Gallbladder - Anatomy, Pathogenesis, and Treatment

Edited by Ahmed ElGeidie

Published in London, United Kingdom

Gallbladder - Anatomy, Pathogenesis, and Treatment
http://dx.doi.org/10.5772/intechopen.1000409
Edited by Ahmed ElGeidie

Contributors
Mazhar Ozkan, Musefa Redwan, Landon Kozai, Larissa Fujii-Lau, Reginald del Pozo, Rohik Anjum, Harshavardhan Panga, Ram Prasad Subedi, Asish Das, Farhanul Huda, Navin Kumar, Carlo de Werra, Antonio Vitiello, Roberto Peltrini, Biancamaria Iacone, Anna Tedesco, Antonio Coppola, Marcello Filotico, Bianca Pacilio, Antonio Gargiulo

First published in London, United Kingdom, 2023 by IntechOpen
IntechOpen is the global imprint of INTECHOPEN LIMITED, registered in England and Wales, registration number: 11086078, 5 Princes Gate Court, London, SW7 2QJ, United Kingdom

British Library Cataloguing-in-Publication Data
A catalogue record for this book is available from the British Library

Additional hard and PDF copies can be obtained from orders@intechopen.com

Gallbladder - Anatomy, Pathogenesis, and Treatment
Edited by Ahmed ElGeidie
p. cm.
Print ISBN 978-1-83769-787-8
Online ISBN 978-1-83769-786-1
eBook (PDF) ISBN 978-1-83769-788-5

Meet the editor

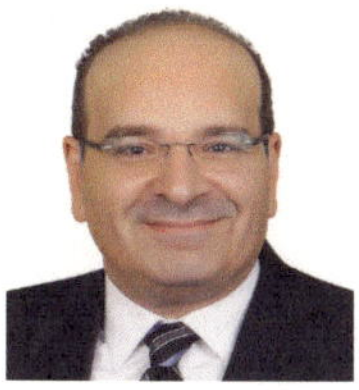

Dr. Ahmed AbdelRaouf ElGeidie has been a professor of general and digestive surgery at Mansoura University, Egypt since 2014. He is the former director of the Gastrointestinal Surgery Center at the same university. He is a board member of the Egyptian Society of Surgeons and a member of the Egyptian committee of promotion of assistant professor in general surgery. Dr. ElGeidie is a peer reviewer for many prestigious surgical journals and an editor of three books on general surgery.

Contents

Preface

Gallbladder disease is highly prevalent and its treatment is controversial. Herein, we provide updated information about gallbladder anatomy, anomalies, pathology, and treatment. Additionally, we discuss endoscopic ultrasound as a new tool in the management of gallbladder disease as well as post-cholecystectomy bile duct injury and gallbladder cancer. Chapters are written by experts in the field from around the world and include figures and illustrations to enhance understanding. I am grateful to the chapter authors for their excellent contributions.

My special thanks go to all who have contributed to this work, particularly the staff at IntechOpen for their assistance throughout the publication process.

I hope readers will find this book a useful resource. More importantly, I hope this work aids medical professionals in their daily practice when dealing with gallbladder disease patients.

Ahmed ElGeidie
Gastrointestinal Surgery Center,
Mansoura University,
Mansoura, Egypt

Chapter 1

The Gallbladder and Extrahepatic Biliary Tract: Anatomy and Variations

Mazhar Ozkan

Abstract

The unusual role of the gallbladder in storing bile, which is crucial for digestive processes and the health of the gastrointestinal tract, sets it apart from other hollow organs. Under the influence of various factors in the gallbladder, where the processes of condensation and reconstitution of bile fluid take place, problems may arise in the cycle and pathologies may appear. Understanding the anatomy of the gallbladder, extrahepatic biliary tract, and surrounding organs is crucial for the diagnosis and treatment of various clinical conditions. The typical and variant anatomy of the gallbladder and the structures surrounding it will be covered in this section.

Keywords: gallbladder, extrahepatic biliary tract, embryological development, anatomy, variation

1. Introduction

Bile is a secretion of water, bile salts, bilirubin, cholesterol, and several electrolytes secreted from the liver and stored in the gallbladder, which plays an important role in the digestion and absorption of fat in the small intestine. Bile is continuously produced in the liver and transported through the bile ducts. It is concentrated while stored in the gallbladder and excreted into the digestive tract with food intake. During these processes, pathological conditions (gallstones, etc.) can occur due to metabolic and other factors (genetic, infection, etc.). Although the ultimate solution is cholecystectomy, removal of the gallbladder, the localization and anatomical variations of the gallbladder, and related formations may cause iatrogenic injuries. This chapter discusses the anatomy and variations of the gallbladder and bile ducts.

2. Development of gallbladder

In humans, the extrahepatic bile ducts and liver develop from the hepatic diverticulum or liver bud, an endodermal outgrowth of the foregut, around the eighteenth day after fertilization (toward the beginning of the fourth week). The gallbladder also develops from the caudal part (pars cystica) of the hepatic foregut diverticulum.

The gallbladder becomes recognizable on the twenty-ninth day after fertilization and the cystic duct around the thirty-fourth day [1]. The gallbladder has a tubular shape until the eleventh week of pregnancy, after which it expands and becomes saccular. The fetal gallbladder is intrahepatic, embedded in the liver fossa [2] until the seventeenth gestational week. It then protrudes under the inferior surface of the liver [3].

The extrahepatic bile ducts develop between the third and eighth embryonic weeks with the extension of the caudal part of the hepatic diverticulum. The extrahepatic parts of the hepatic duct and the right and left hepatic ducts develop from the cranial part of the hepatic diverticulum (pars hepatica). The proximal parts of the hilar ducts originate from the intrahepatic ductal plates. At the beginning of the fifth gestational week, the hepatobiliary anatomical structures (gallbladder, cystic duct, hepatic ducts, common bile duct, and ventral pancreas) are in the ventral mesentery of the duodenum. At the end of the fifth week, with the rotation of the duodenum to the right side, the developing common bile duct is displaced to its new position in the dorsal part of the duodenum. The lower part of the common bile duct and the ventral pancreatic primordium enter the dorsal mesentery and join the dorsal pancreatic primordium. They become secondary retroperitoneal, located anterior to the retroperitoneal organs. The fusion fascia surrounding these structures contributes to the formation of the anterior layer of Gerota's fascia.

In the sixth gestational week, the developing extrahepatic biliary tract is organized. By the seventh week, the lumen reaches the cystic duct, but the gallbladder is still a cluster of cells (until the twelfth week). Abnormalities during the reorganization of the extrahepatic biliary tract can affect the development of the bile ducts and gallbladder, resulting in various types of atresia. In addition, two or more lumens may be present in the duct, and duplications may occur due to their inability to merge. In the ninth week, the muscular part of the gallbladder develops from the mesenchymal cells surrounding the epithelial primordium.

An outward growth from the common bile duct forms the ventral pancreas. The connection of the common bile duct with the anterior intestine occurs at the major duodenal papilla in the second part of the duodenum. Here, the terminal part of the common bile duct and the terminal part of the pancreatic duct come together to form a short duct.

Other associated anomalies include annular pancreas, malrotation, duodenal atresia, imperforate anus, portal and inferior vena cava abnormalities, polysplenia, congenital heart disease, and urinary tract anomalies. It has been reported that reovirus type-3 infections may lead to possible biliary atresia.

Agenesis of the gallbladder is extremely rare. It may be associated with normal or atresia biliary tract. One in six patients with extrahepatic biliary atresia has gallbladder agenesis. The rapid growth of the liver in the second gestational month is important to understand anomalies related to the localization of the gallbladder. Positional anomalies of the gallbladder are intrahepatic, retrohepatic, left-sided, and ptotic (hanging).

The retrohepatic gallbladder is thought to be associated with the abnormal migration of the gallbladder-cystic duct bud posteriorly.

Left-sided gallbladder occurs rarely and can be found on the undersurface of the left lobe of the liver or to the left of the falciform ligament. It may have a cystic duct with a normal position, or it may angulate sharply to the left.

In the twelfth week, the gallbladder becomes hollow by vacuolization. Errors in vacuolization can lead to septation within the gallbladder. The presence of a complete septation is referred to as gallbladder duplication. Duplication can occur at various levels. When the fundus and corpus are involved starting from the neck, it is called external duplication. In a mild type, a duplication may occur that is not visible externally but is completely separated internally by a longitudinal septum. Partial duplications can also occur due to gallbladder-cystic duct bifurcation. In this case, duplications of the cystic duct or gallbladder (as two separate sacs) may occur.

Embryologic changes in the terminal part of the gallbladder-cystic duct bud can cause deformities such as Phrygian cap, hourglass gallbladder, Hartmann's pouch, and diverticula. Some of these may be acquired rather than congenital (e.g., Hartmann's pouch may occur as a result of dilatation of the infundibulum due to chronic obstruction).

The gallbladder, because of its solid structure, is not sonographically distinguishable until the second trimester of pregnancy. Around the twentieth gestational week, it can be identified in 65% of fetuses [4].

3. Anatomy of gallbladder

The gallbladder is a flask- or pear-shaped diverticulum connected to the extrahepatic bile duct by a duct called the ductus cysticus. It has three parts: fundus, corpus, and neck (**Figure 1**). It is involved in the storage, concentration, and rehydration of bile from hepatocytes and its ejection into the digestive tract. This function is regulated by the parasympathetic nervous system and hormones, especially cholecystokinin.

In the living organism, it is gray-blue in color and is located in a depression (fossa vesicae biliaris) on the visceral surface of the right lobe of the liver (segments IV and V)

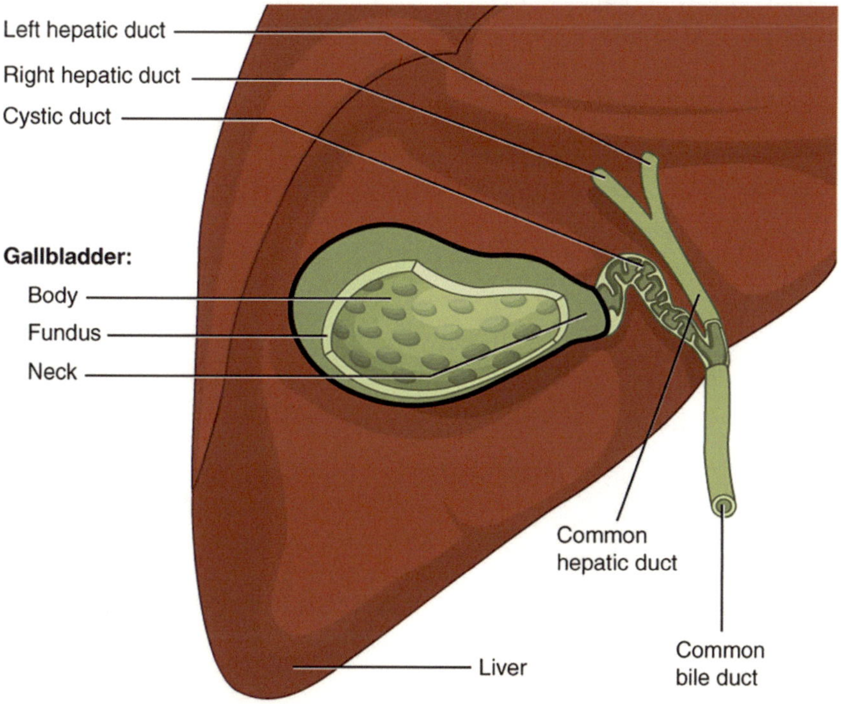

Figure 1.
Anatomy and location of the gallbladder [5].

and is fixed to it by the visceral peritoneum. This fossa is located at the caudal border of the interlobar fissure, an embryologic structure separating the right and left hepatic lobes. Within this fissure (fissure of Gans, Rouviere's sulcus, or incisura hepatis dextra) is the middle hepatic vein. It is a useful anatomic landmark in hepatic resection and laparoscopic cholecystectomy (the cystic duct and artery are located anterosuperior to the sulcus, whereas the common bile duct is posteroinferior) [5]. In the posterosuperior part of the fossa is the porta hepatis through which the hepatic artery, portal vein, and common bile duct pass. The peritoneum surrounds these structures and is called the hepatoduodenal ligament (free edge of the lesser omentum, **Figure 2**). A fold extending from the hepatoduodenal ligament around the gallbladder is called the cholecystoduodenal ligament.

In an adult, the gallbladder is 7 to 10 cm long and has a volume of 25 (resting/empty) to 50 ml [7]. The relationship of the gallbladder to the liver varies and has been classified into seven groups by [8]. Outside of these groups, the gallbladder may very rarely be surrounded by the parenchyma of the liver (intrahepatic gallbladder) [9]. In cases that allow the gallbladder to move away from the liver, more caution should be exercised as there is a risk of gallbladder torsion [10, 11].

In most of the population (approximately 75% according to Tihan [8]), the gallbladder has a fundus that contacts the anterior abdominal wall in the transpyloric plane, a corpus located in the fossa, and a neck located most medially. The junction of the fundus and corpus is the widest part of the gallbladder and narrows toward the neck. The most rapidly narrowing part is called the infundibulum. The collum vesicae biliaris is close to the porta hepatis and is attached to the liver by a short and thin peritoneal attachment (mesentery). This peritoneal attachment usually contains the cystic artery. The mesenteric attachment shortens as it moves from the neck to the body and covers the gallbladder fossa. The mucosa on the inner wall of the neck contains oblique folds, which are continuous with the spiral mucosal folds in the cystic duct [12]. The neck of the gallbladder expands laterally to form the body. The

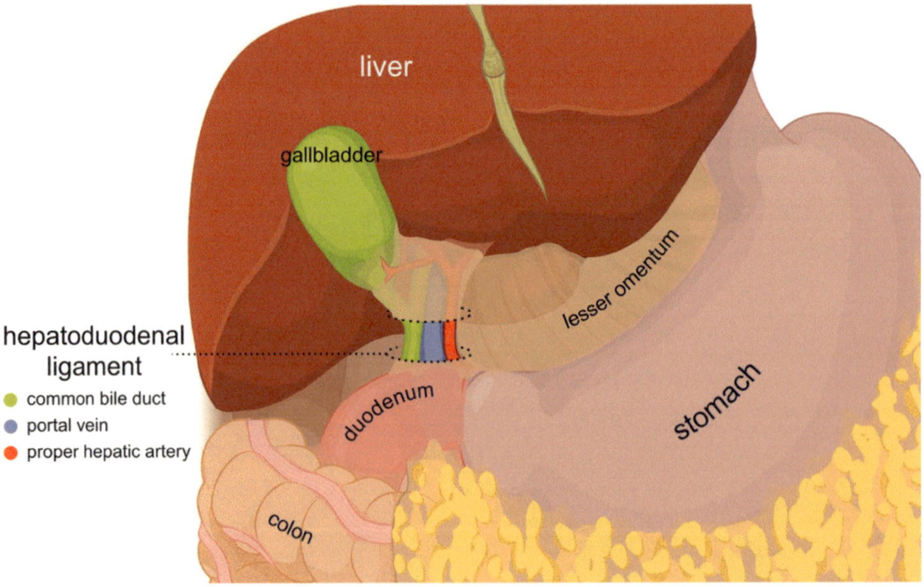

Figure 2.
The hepatoduodenal ligament and its contents [6].

expansion site is associated with gallstone disease and is called "Hartmann's pouch." The neck of the gallbladder is located in front of the descending part, the second part of the duodenum.

The bulbous fundus of the gallbladder is located at the lateral end of the corpus and usually crosses the inferior margin of the liver and contacts the parietal peritoneum on the abdominal wall behind the ninth costal cartilage, at the lateral edge of the right rectus abdominis. This area is examined in the clinical examination of gallbladder enlargement. The gallbladder is posteroinferiorly adjacent to the duodenum as well as the transverse colon and sometimes the inferior vena cava.

The gallbladder is usually supplied by the cystic artery branching from the right hepatic artery. Venous drainage occurs *via* numerous, small, unnamed veins to the portal venous system. Lymphatic drainage occurs to the lymph nodes in the porta hepatis and then to the preaortic lymph nodes in the celiac axis.

The gallbladder is histologically composed of three layers. The outermost serous layer is formed by the peritoneum and is usually lost where the gallbladder contacts the liver and is replaced by a connective tissue. Microscopic bile ductules (radicles, ducts of Luschka) may extend from the intrahepatic bile ducts into this connective tissue. The innermost mucosal layer consists of columnar epithelium and has both absorption and mucus-secretory functions. The inner surface of the gallbladder is surrounded by thin folds that become prominent during contraction. The mucosa protrudes into the outer layers in sacs, forming the Rokitansky-Aschoff sinuses. These can be associated with disease and are found in most adults. The mucosa of the gallbladder is continuous with the mucosa of the cystic duct. The mucosa is lifted by spiral folds (Heister valves). The intervening muscular layer comprises circular, longitudinal, and obliquely oriented muscle fibers and surrounding connective tissue. The muscular layer also continues in the wall of the cystic duct but not in the wall of the bile ducts.

The size and shape of the gallbladder is variable. The fundus may be elongated and highly mobile. Rarely, the fundus curves over the corpus and is called a Phrygian cap, which may be misinterpreted on ultrasonographic examination as the presence of a septum. Other variations of the gallbladder include agenesis, duplication, the presence of double cystic duct, internal septation, and ectopic localization [13]. Boyden [14] and Harlaftis et al. classified gallbladder variations as Type 1 and Type 2, which were further subdivided (**Figure 3**) [15, 16]

Although variations of the gallbladder are rare, they are very important in patients requiring surgery for gallbladder diseases or gallstones [17, 18].

4. Intrahepatic biliary tract

The left half of the liver has segmental ducts with a relatively constant pattern, and one segmental duct can drain more than one segment. The left hepatic duct is formed by the fusion of segment II and segment III ducts and is located posterior or to the left of the umbilical portion of the left portal vein. Bile drainage of segment IV varies but is accomplished by a single duct that opens into the left hepatic duct. The right hepatic duct is formed by the union of the right anterior (medial) and posterior (lateral) sectoral ducts. The right anterior (medial) sectoral duct drains segments V and VIII, and the right posterior (lateral) sectoral duct drains segments VI and VII. The right posterior sectoral duct usually bends on the posterior aspect of the right anterior duct and converges medially. This is called Hjortsö's crook and is an important condition to be considered during liver resection.

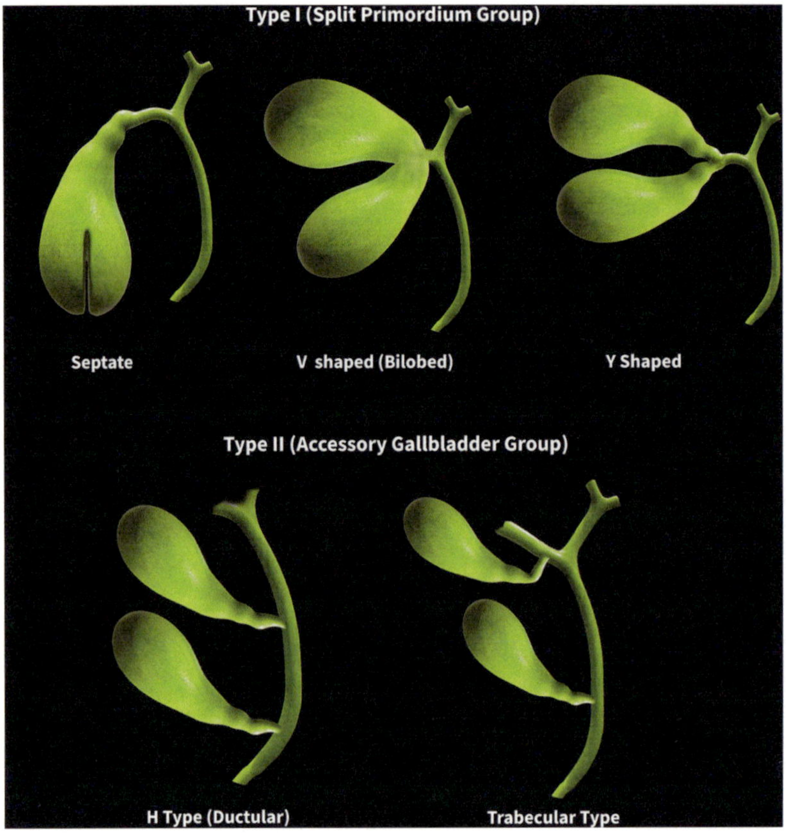

Figure 3.
Variations of the gallbladder.

The right hepatic duct and its branches show more variations than the left ductal system [19]. They are divided into six main groups. Left intrahepatic ductal variations are mostly related to the drainage pattern of segment IV. This segmental duct usually drains into the left hepatic duct but can sometimes open into the segment II or even III duct, the right anterior sectoral duct, or even the common hepatic duct [20].

A bile duct from segment V of the liver, described by Luschka, may pass through the fossa of the gallbladder and open into the right hepatic duct or its anterior sectoral branch, the common hepatic duct, or, rarely, the cystic duct. These ducts, classified as Luschka's ducts, occur in 30% of the population in various sizes, whereas ducts 1 to 2 mm in diameter have a prevalence of only 5% [21]. Damage to these variational ducts during cholecystectomy can cause postoperative complications such as bile leakage.

5. Extrahepatic biliary tract

After leaving the liver, the right and left hepatic ducts merge at the right edge of the porta hepatis to form the common hepatic duct (**Figure 4**). The extrahepatic right duct is short (0.5 to 2.0 cm in adults) and vertically oriented. The extrahepatic left duct is longer (1.5 to 3.5 cm) and more horizontal, lying on the inferior margin of segment IV. Access to the extrahepatic segment of the left hepatic duct is important during surgical biliary bypass for benign hilar bile duct strictures.

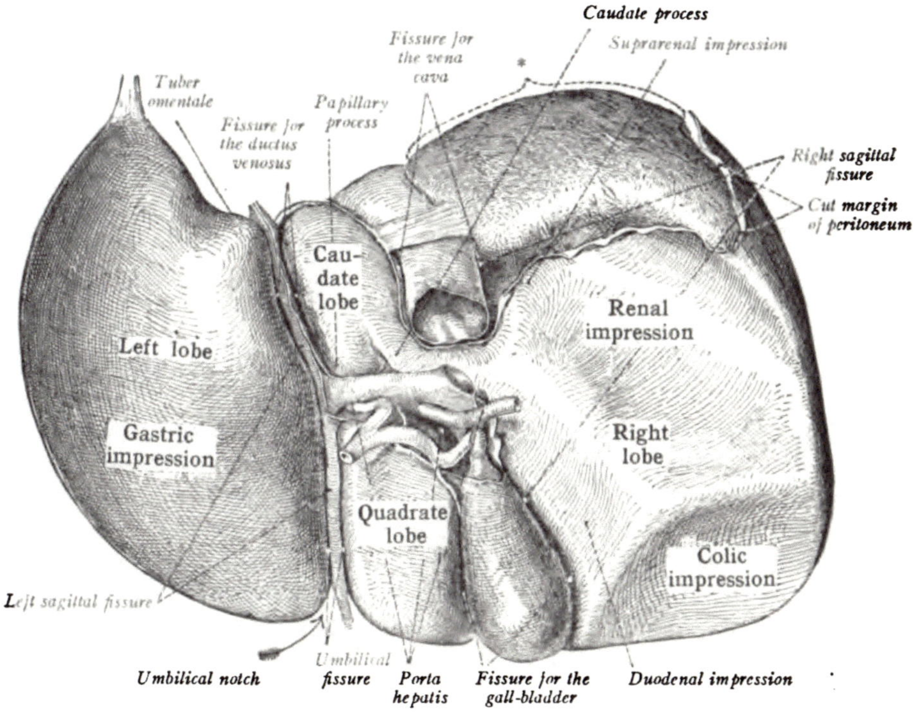

Figure 4.
Porta hepatis and its content [22].

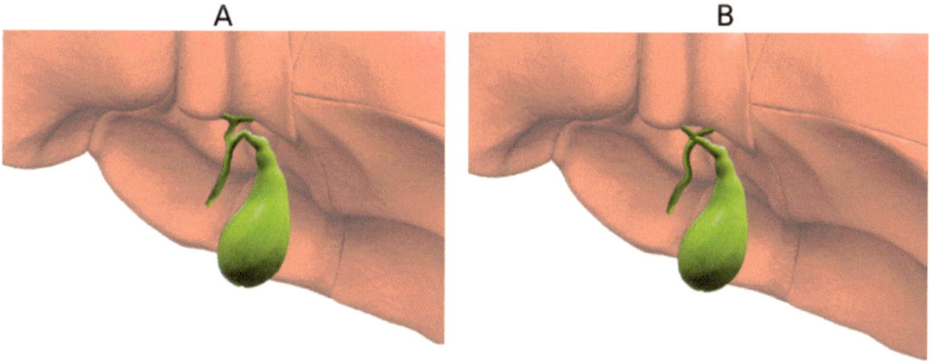

Figure 5.
Formation of the common hepatic duct. A: normal case; B: cystohepatic junction with aberrant common hepatic duct formation.

After leaving the liver, the right and left hepatic ducts merge 2.5 to 25 mm from the liver parenchyma to form the common hepatic duct. The left hepatic duct has a longer extrahepatic course than the right hepatic duct (17 and 9 mm, respectively). In some cases, the junction may remain within the liver parenchyma as the liver enlarges. The length of the common hepatic duct can vary considerably (15 to 35 mm). Sometimes, the cystic duct may open at the junction of the right and left hepatic ducts to form the common bile duct (**Figure 5B**). Three types of cystohepatic junction have been classified as angular, parallel, and spiral.

In adults, the common hepatic duct is 3 cm long and is obliquely joined to the cystic duct on the right side and is called the common bile duct. The common hepatic duct is located to the right of the hepatic artery and anterior to the portal vein within the hepatoduodenal ligament. In adults, the normal common hepatic duct lumen diameter is less than 5 mm in ultrasound measurements.

The cystic duct drains the gallbladder into the common bile duct (**Figure 6**). It has a length of 2 to 4 cm and a lumen diameter of 2 to 3 mm in adults [12]. With its tortuous structure, it passes through the posterior and medial part of the neck of the gallbladder, merges with the common hepatic duct, and forms the common bile duct. The junction of the cystic duct with the common hepatic duct varies. In most people, it opens into the middle third of the total length of the common hepatic and common bile ducts, but it may open more distally or more proximally (into the common hepatic duct or the right hepatic duct). It usually opens to the medial surface of the common hepatic duct but may also join medially, anteriorly, or posteriorly.

The cystic duct usually forms an oblique angle at its junction with the common hepatic duct, but sometimes it may make a spiral turn around it, or it may descend parallel to it for a while and merge within the hepatoduodenal ligament.

The cystic duct may rarely be double or absent or may take an abnormal hepatic duct from segment V of the liver. These variations are very important for surgical interventions such as cholecystectomy, and in cases where the anatomy is not clear enough, it is important to detect them with a cholangiogram before the operation. The cystic duct should be occluded away from the common bile duct during cholecystectomy without damaging the common bile duct.

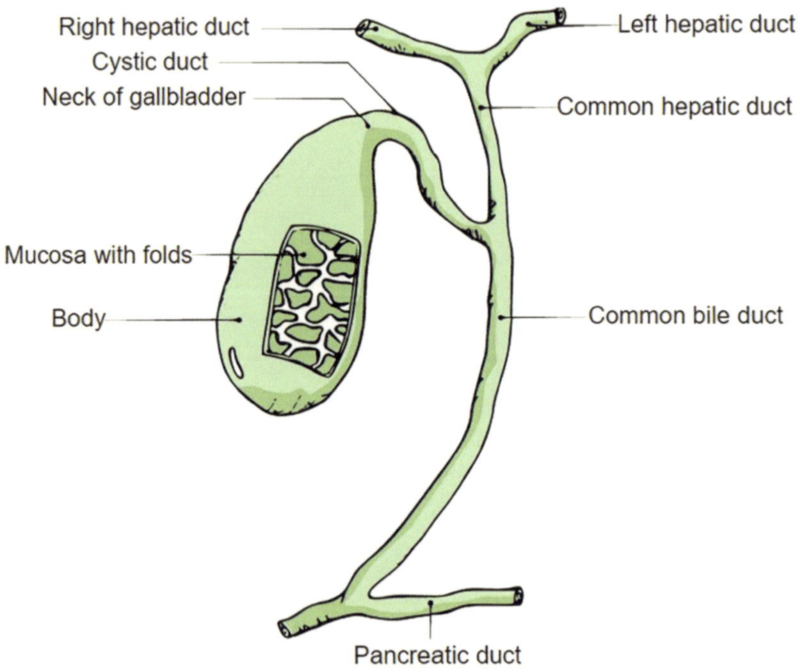

Figure 6.
Extrahepatic biliary tract anatomy [23].

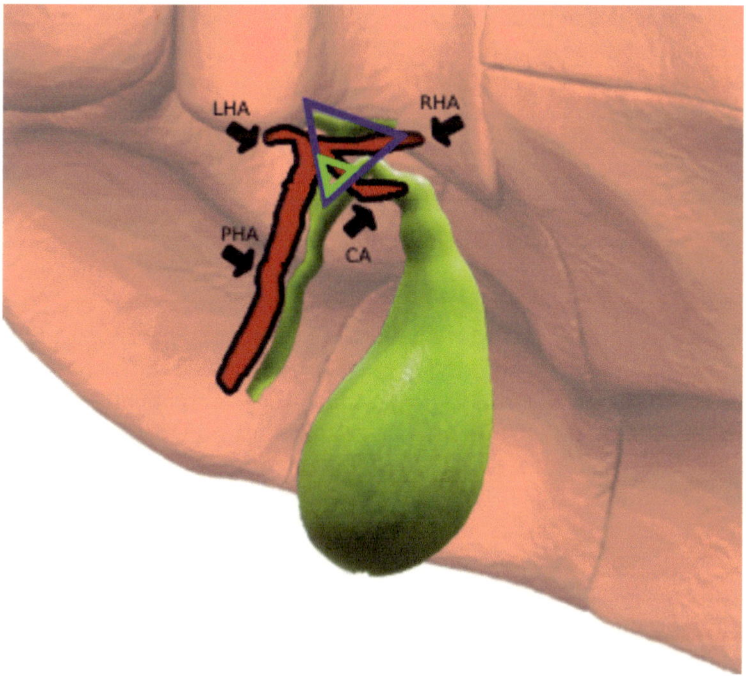

Figure 7.
Hepatobiliary (blue) and Calot's (green) triangles. LHA, left hepatic artery; RHA, right hepatic artery; PHA, proper hepatic artery; CA, cystic artery.

The triangular area formed by the cystic duct, the common hepatic duct, and the lower surface of the liver is called the hepatobiliary triangle (**Figure 7**, blue triangle). This triangle is often confused with Calot's triangle (**Figure 7**, green triangle), an isosceles triangle with the common hepatic duct forming the base and the cystic artery and cystic duct forming the sides [24]. The hepatobiliary triangle is bridged by a two-layered peritoneum that forms the short and diverse mesentery of the cystic duct. Between the two sheets of the peritoneum are various amounts of adipose tissue, lymph vessels, cystic lymph node, autonomic nerves, and the cystic artery, which usually extends from the right hepatic artery to the gallbladder. Sometimes, an accessory bile duct can also be seen here. A good understanding of the anatomy of the biliary or arterial structures involved in the structure of the triangle is crucial to preventing damage to the common hepatic duct, common bile duct, or right hepatic artery during cholecystectomy [25, 26].

The common bile duct is formed close to the porta hepatis by the union of the cystic duct and the common hepatic duct. In adults, the duct is usually 6 to 8 cm in length, with a luminal diameter of less than 7 mm measured by ultrasound [27]. The diameter changes with age (3.6 mm under 60 years, 4 mm over 80 years). The common bile duct can be divided into three segments: supraduodenal, retroduodenal, and pancreatic segments. The supraduodenal segment descends posteriorly and slightly to the left, anterior to the epiploic foramen and inferior vena cava, to the right of the hepatic artery on the free right margin of the lesser omentum, and to the right-anterior to the portal vein. This segment is the most surgically accessible part of the common bile duct. The retroduodenal segment is located behind the first part of the duodenum to the right of the gastroduodenal artery. The pancreatic segment lies in a groove behind the head of the pancreas. Here, it is embedded in the gland to varying degrees. It runs in front of the right renal vein 2 cm from the second part of the duodenum. The posterior superior pancreaticoduodenal branch of the gastroduodenal artery descends anterior to the retroduodenal portion of the common bile duct. When it crosses the upper edge of the pancreas, the artery winds around the common bile duct.

The common bile duct runs down and medially behind the head of the pancreas, approaching the medial end of the main pancreatic duct. Together, the two ducts enter the wall of the second part of the duodenum and form a short duct, 2 to 10 mm long. This duct opens into the medial wall of the second part of the duodenum through the major duodenal papilla after an expansion called the hepatopancreatic ampulla (of Vater). Clinically, this region is called the pancreaticobiliary junction. Sometimes, the two ducts may merge before entering the duodenum to form a long common duct, but sometimes, they resist the duodenum separated from each other by a septum (**Figure 8**).

In the terminal 5 to 10 mm of the common bile duct and main pancreatic duct, the mucosa has plicae with a complex circular organization. Their distribution and orientation are known to prevent the reflux of duodenal contents into the ducts and cause difficulty in the cannulation of the major duodenal papilla during endoscopic retrograde cholangiopancreatography (ERCP).

The common bile duct (bile duct sphincter), the main pancreatic duct (pancreatic duct sphincter), and the hepatopancreatic ampulla (sphincter of Oddi) are surrounded by complexly organized circular smooth muscle fibers. This sphincter muscle complex is 15 to 20 mm in length and is located within the duodenal wall but is anatomically and developmentally separate from the surrounding duodenal muscle fibers. The sphincter complex regulates the passage of pancreatic secretions and bile into the duodenum and prevents the reflux of duodenal contents into the ductal

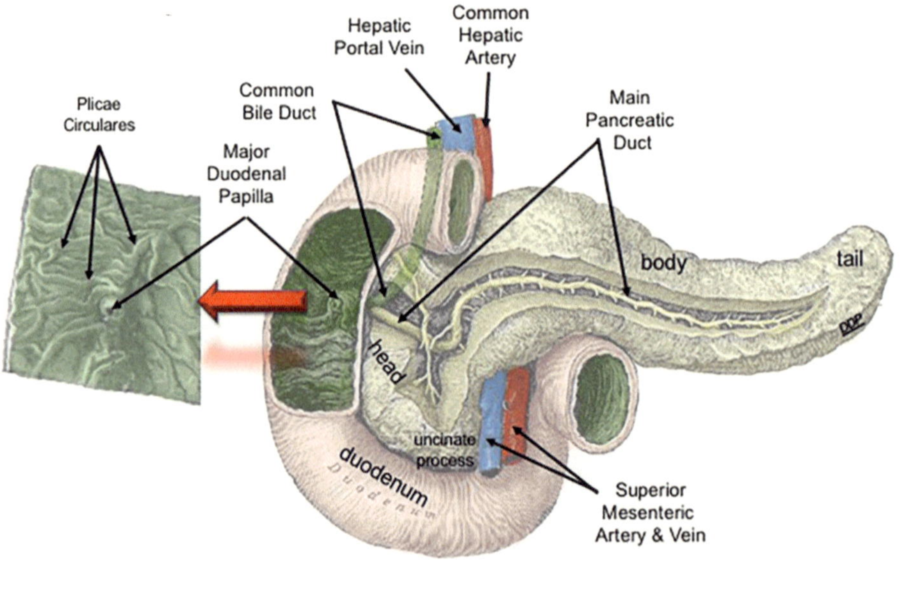

Figure 8.
Common bile duct and duodenum [28].

system. Cholecystokinin (CKK) inhibits the sphincter and causes contraction of the gallbladder. During ERCP, it may be necessary to divide the upper part of the sphincter of Oddi (sphincterotomy) to access the common bile duct. The pancreaticobiliary connection can be affected by various congenital and acquired diseases. An abnormal junction of the bile and pancreatic ducts can lead to congenital bile duct dilatation, recurrent pancreatitis, and/or gallbladder cancers. Gallstone obstructions and periampullary tumors are pathologies that can occur later.

The innervation of the gallbladder and extrahepatic biliary tract is mediated by branches from the hepatic plexus. Parasympathetic fibers from the vagus nerve as well as CKK cause contractions of the gallbladder. Postganglionic sympathetic fibers from the coeliac and superior mesenteric ganglia cause inhibition of the smooth muscles of the gallbladder. On the other hand, these sympathetic fibers receive the pain sensation of the gallbladder and carry it to the seventh and ninth (T7–T9) spinal cord segments *via* the central extensions of the neurons forming the greater and lesser splanchnic nerves. Visceral pain of the gallbladder radiates to the right hypochondrium and epigastrium and may be felt in the back below the right scapula. Involvement of the parietal peritoneum surrounding the gallbladder causes localized pain in the right upper quadrant.

Lymphatic drainage of the gallbladder and cystic duct occurs first to the cystic node above the cystic duct in the hepatobiliary triangle, then to the lymph nodes at the free edge of the lesser omentum, and then to the coeliac lymph nodes along the common hepatic artery. Some lymph also drains around the common bile duct to the superior pancreaticoduodenal node, which is connected to the para-aortic nodes, and to the superior mesenteric lymph nodes. Lymph from the part of the gallbladder adjacent to the liver passes into the intrahepatic lymph vessels [29].

6. Conclusion

Changing lifestyles and diets have led to an increase in clinical conditions related to the gallbladder and biliary tract. Since gallstone-related disorders affect the main pancreatic duct as well as the bile ducts, cholecystectomy gains importance as a permanent and effective solution. A good knowledge of the anatomy of the gallbladder and bile ducts is essential for a successful and uncomplicated surgery. In addition to basic knowledge of the anatomy of the biliary tract, intraoperative evaluation prevents possible injuries [30, 31]. The advantages of laparoscopic cholecystectomy such as minimal intervention and rapid recovery are limited by the complications that may be caused by anatomic variations. Therefore, both surgical intervention and the development of new treatment modalities can only be possible by transferring the current knowledge in the most accurate and broadest way.

Author details

Mazhar Ozkan
Anatomy Department, School of Medicine, Tekirdag Namik Kemal University, Tekirdag, Turkiye

*Address all correspondence to: ozkanmazhar@gmail.com

References

[1] Roskams T, Desmet V. Embryology of extra- and intrahepatic bile ducts, the ductal plate. Anatomical Record (Hoboken, N.J.: 2007). 2008;**291**(6): 628-635. DOI: 10.1002/ar.20710

[2] Wang BJ, Kim JH, Yu HC, Rodríguez-Vázquez JF, Murakami G, Cho BH. Fetal intrahepatic gallbladder and topographical anatomy of the liver hilar region and hepatocystic triangle. Clinical Anatomy (New York, NY). 2012;**25**(5):619-627. DOI: 10.1002/ca.21288

[3] Haffajee MR. The fetal gallbladder: morphology and morphometry by microdissection. Surgical and Radiologic Anatomy. 2000;**22**(5-6):261-270. DOI: 10.1007/s00276-000-0261-6

[4] Meilstrup JW. Imaging Atlas of the Normal Gallbladder and Its Variants. CRC Press; 2018

[5] Dahmane R, Morjane A, Starc A. Anatomy and surgical relevance of Rouviere's sulcus. ScientificWorldJournal. 2013;**2013**:254287. DOI: 10.1155/2013/254287

[6] Remesz O. Hepatoduodenal ligament. [Online]. Accessed date: https://upload.wikimedia.org/wikipedia/commons/4/44/Hepatoduodenal_ligament_EN.svg

[7] Di Ciaula A, Wang DQ-H, Portincasa P. Gallbladder and gastric motility in obese newborns, pre-adolescents and adults. Journal of Gastroenterology and Hepatology. 2012;**27**(8):1298-1305. DOI: 10.1111/j.1440-1746.2012.07149.x

[8] Tihan D et al. The effect of morphometric and anatomic relationship of gallbladder to the liver on standard laparoscopic cholecystectomies and proposal of a new anatomical classification. European Review for Medical and Pharmacological Sciences. 2016;**20**(8):1458-1466

[9] Guiteau JJ, Fisher M, Cotton RT, Goss JA. Intrahepatic gallbladder. Journal of the American College of Surgeons. 2009;**209, 5**:s. 672. DOI: 10.1016/j.jamcollsurg.2009.03.027

[10] Ashaolu JO, Ukwenya VO, Adenowo TK. Cystoduodenal ligament as an abnormal fold and the accompanying anatomical and clinical implications. Surgical and Radiologic Anatomy. 2011;**33**(2):171-174. DOI: 10.1007/s00276-010-0736-z

[11] Gupta V, Singh V, Sewkani A, Purohit D, Varshney R, Varshney S. Torsion of gall bladder, a rare entity: a case report and review article. Cases Journal. 2009;**2**:193. DOI: 10.1186/1757-1626-2-193

[12] Dasgupta D, Stringer MD. Cystic duct and Heister's 'valves'. Clinical Anatomy (New York, NY). 2005;**18**(2):81-87. DOI: 10.1002/ca.20118

[13] Faure JP, Doucet C, Scepi M, Rigoard P, Carretier M, Richer JP. Abnormalities of the gallbladder, clinical effects. Surgical and Radiologic Anatomy. 2008;**30**(4):285-290. DOI: 10.1007/s00276-008-0332-7

[14] Boyden EA. The accessory gallbladder an embryological and comparative study of aberrant biliary vesicles occurring in man and the domestic mammals. American Journal of Anatomy. 1926;**38**(2):177-231

[15] Harlaftis N, Gray SW, Skandalakis JE. Multiple gallbladders. Surgery, Gynecology & Obstetrics. 1977;**145**(6):928-934

[16] Botsford A, McKay K, Hartery A, Hapgood C. MRCP imaging of duplicate gallbladder: A case report and review of the literature. Surgical and Radiologic Anatomy. 2015;**37**(5):425-429. DOI: 10.1007/s00276-015-1456-1

[17] Castorina S, Scilletta R, Domergue J. Gallbladder agenesis: Laparoscopic views of a significant diagnostic challenge. Surgical and Radiologic Anatomy. 2014;**36**(6):619-620. DOI: 10.1007/s00276-014-1263-0

[18] Singh B, Ramsaroop L, Allopi L, Moodley J, Satyapal KS. Duplicate gallbladder: An unusual case report. Surgical and Radiologic Anatomy. 2006;**28**(6):654-657. DOI: 10.1007/s00276-006-0139-3

[19] Cucchetti A et al. Anatomic variations of intrahepatic bile ducts in a European series and meta-analysis of the literature. Journal of Gastrointestinal Surgery. 2011;**15**(4):623-630. DOI: 10.1007/s11605-011-1447-4

[20] Chaib E, Kanas AF, Galvão FHF, D'Albuquerque LAC. Bile duct confluence: Anatomic variations and its classification. Surgical and Radiologic Anatomy. 2014;**36**(2):105-109. DOI: 10.1007/s00276-013-1157-6

[21] Ko K et al. A study of the subvesical bile duct (duct of Luschka) in resected liver specimens. World Journal of Surgery. 2006;**30**(7):1316-1320. DOI: 10.1007/s00268-005-0469-z

[22] Sobotta J. An anatomical illustration from the 1906 edition of Sobotta's Atlas and Text-book of Human Anatomy with English terminology

[23] LukesAnatomy. Gross Gallbladder anatomy and local ducts. [Online]. Accessed date: https://upload.wikimedia.org/wikipedia/commons/6/61/GallbladderAnatomy.png

[24] Stringer MD. Gallbladder and Extrahepatic Bile Ducts. In: Tubbs RS, Shoja MM, Loukas M, editors. Bergman's Comprehensive Encyclopedia of Human Anatomic Variation. 2016. DOI: 10.1002/9781118430309.ch107

[25] Suzuki M, Akaishi S, Rikiyama T, Naitoh T, Rahman MM, Matsuno S. Laparoscopic cholecystectomy, Calot's triangle, and variations in cystic arterial supply. Surgical Endoscopy. 2000;**14**(2):141-144. DOI: 10.1007/s004649900086

[26] Talpur KAH, Laghari AA, Yousfani SA, Malik AM, Memon AI, Khan SA. Anatomical variations and congenital anomalies of extra hepatic biliary system encountered during laparoscopic cholecystectomy. JPMA. Journal of the Pakistan Medical Association. 2010;**60**(2):89-93

[27] Perret RS, Sloop GD, Borne JA. Common bile duct measurements in an elderly population. Journal of Ultrasound in Medicine. 2000;**19**(11):727-730; quiz 731. DOI: 10.7863/jum.2000.19.11.727

[28] Cypressvine, PancreasColor.jpg. [Online]. Accessed date: https://commons.wikimedia.org/wiki/File:PancreasColor.jpg

[29] Sato T, Ito M, Sakamoto H. Pictorial dissection review of the lymphatic pathways from the gallbladder to the abdominal para-aortic lymph nodes and their relationships to the surrounding structures. Surgical and Radiologic Anatomy. 2013;**35**(7):615-621. DOI: 10.1007/s00276-013-1088-2

[30] Buddingh KT, Nieuwenhuijs VB, van Buuren L, Hulscher JBF, de Jong JS, van Dam GM. Intraoperative assessment of biliary anatomy for prevention of bile duct injury: A review of current and future patient safety interventions. Surgical Endoscopy. 2011;**25**(8):2449-2461. DOI: 10.1007/s00464-011-1639-8

[31] Brunt LM et al. Safe Cholecystectomy Multi-society Practice Guideline and State of the Art Consensus Conference on Prevention of Bile Duct Injury During Cholecystectomy. Annals of Surgery. 2020;**272**(1):3-23. DOI: 10.1097/SLA.0000000000003791

Chapter 2

Gallbladder Position Anomalies: Clinical Impacts and Management

Musefa Redwan

Abstract

Gallbladder position anomalies are rare. Normally, the gallbladder is located at the inferior surface of the right lobe of the liver between segments IV and V, covered by the peritoneum, and attached to the liver by its mesentery in the gall bladder fossa. Any position other than this is defined as a gallbladder position anomaly. Gallbladder ectopia variants may include floating, intrahepatic, retroperitoneal, and left-sided gallbladder, among others. According to some literature, floating gallbladder is the most common among these anomalies, occurring in 4.6% of population; however, there is no clear and adequate data on incidence and variants of gallbladder position anomalies. Because of their rare occurrence and lack of specific clinical and imaging features, their possible presence and clinical sequelae are not usually considered in clinical practice. This results in delayed diagnosis and treatment of sequelae, such as in gallbladder volvulus (GBV). Similarly, gallbladder position and associated biliary tree and vascular anomalies should be identified during the preoperative period. Failing to do this may have devastating outcomes. Though clinical impacts and management of gallbladder position anomalies are explained in some literature, they are not well covered by most of the currently available surgical books. To fill this gap, this chapter discusses the embryology, variants, prevalence, clinical impacts, and management of ectopic gallbladder as well as ways to increase the rate of preoperative diagnosis and methods to decrease adverse outcomes and morbidity.

Keywords: gallbladder position anomalies, gallbladder malpositions, gallbladder ectopia, gallbladder volvulus, gallbladder hernia, laparoscopic cholecystectomy

1. Introduction

Gallbladder position anomalies are rare [1, 2]. Normally, the gallbladder is located at the inferior surface of the right lobe of the liver between hepatic segments IV and V. It is covered by the peritoneum and adhered to the liver by its mesentery in gall bladder fossa at cantle's line to the right of the falciform ligament. Any position other than this is defined as gallbladder malposition [2, 3]. Gallbladder ectopia variants may include floating, intrahepatic, retroperitoneal, and left-sided gallbladder [2, 4]. According to some literature, floating gallbladder is the most common among these anomalies, occurring in 4.6% of population [5]; however, there is no clear and adequate data on incidence and variants of gallbladder position anomalies [1–4, 6]. Floating gallbladder may result in volvulus in the presence of precipitating factors [5, 7]. The clinical impacts of ectopic gallbladder include [8]:

IntechOpen

misdiagnosis of common gallbladder pathologies due to malposition or misdiagnosis of gallbladder volvulus (GBV) as acute cholecystitis

- confusion in interpretation of diagnostic imaging
- associated biliary tree and vascular anomalies
- technical difficulties during surgery

Because of their rare occurrence as well as lack of specific clinical and imaging features, the possible presence and clinical sequelae of gallbladder position anomalies are not usually considered in clinical practice. This results in delayed diagnosis and treatment of sequelae, as in GBV [6, 7]. Gallbladder position and associated biliary tree and vascular anomalies should be identified preoperatively. Failing to do so may have devastating outcomes, such as biliary duct injury or major vascular injury with hepatic necrosis. Even though preoperative diagnosis of position anomalies is possible with magnetic resonance cholangiopancreatography (MRCP), most are still being diagnosed intraoperatively. Adequate knowledge of these anatomical variants of the gallbladder will help modify techniques like laparoscopic cholecystectomy and prevent injury in the presence of biliary tree and vascular anomalies. This chapter reviews gallbladder embryology, anatomy, position anomaly variants, pathogenesis, clinical significance, and treatment.

2. Anatomy and embryology of the biliary system

2.1 Embryology of the biliary tree

The hepatobiliary system develops as an endodermal outgrowth from the ventral surface of the distal fore gut when the embryo is 3 mm in size (approximately 4th week of gestation) (**Figure 1A**). This outgrowth is called the hepatic

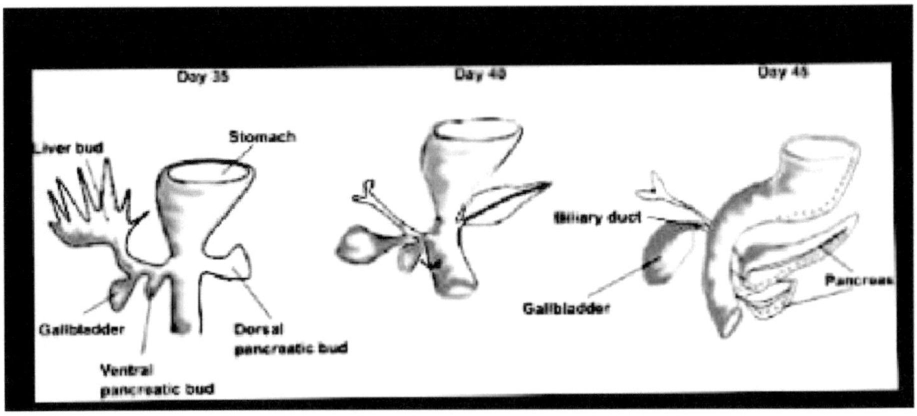

Figure 1.
Hepato biliary system development. A. At 5th week of development showimg cranial & caudal hepatic buds. (taken from Sahu and Yang) [9].

diverticulum. With further proliferation, when the embryo is 5 mm in size (approximately early 5th week of gestation), the hepatic diverticulum divides into larger cranial and smaller caudal buds. The cranial bud is called pars hepatica, which will differentiate into liver and intrahepatic ducts, and the caudal bud is called pars cystica, which will further differentiate into superior and inferior buds. The superior bud differentiated gallbladder and the cystic duct and inferior bud gives ventral pancreas (**Figure 1B**). At about 32 days of gestation, the primordial gallbladder and common bile duct (CBD) appear. When the embryo is 7–9 mm (approximately 6th week of gestation), the gallbladder and cystic duct emerge and connect with the CBD, forming the liver and intrahepatic ducts. Bile starts to drain to the duodenum when the embryo is 12 mm (8th week of gestation). Initially, the gallbladder precursor attaches to the ventral surface of the duodenal precursor, with differential growth rotation to the right occurring at this stage bringing about attachment to the dorsal aspect of the duodenum. This results in the gallbladder precursor lying at the free edge of the ventral mesentery. Further differential growth makes the gallbladder migrate to the anterior inferior surface of the right hepatic lobe where it become intrahepatic. At 12 mm (approximately 8th week of gestation), the gallbladder migrates, becomes extrahepatic, and attaches to the anterior inferior surface of the liver between hepatic segments IV and V. The ventral mesentery that lies between the liver and foregut will develop into a gastrohepatic and hepatoduodenal ligament. That lies between Liver & anterior abdominal wall will persist as falcifarum ligament, contains obliterated umbilical vein (ligamentum teres) in its free edge. When the embryo is 6 mm in size (approximately early 5th week of gestation), the developing liver is supplied by two blood vessels: the right and left umbilical veins. The left umbilical vein becomes one of the afferent vessels to the liver, but the right umbilical vein atrophies when the embryo is 7 mm (at the end of 5th week of gestation). The left umbilical vein is later obliterated and becomes the falciform ligament, and the typical umbilical portion of the main portal vein is formed [9, 10].

If any disruption occurs during migration, gallbladder position variations may occur.

1. If any disruption occurs during gallbladder migration from the free edge of the ventral mesentery to the right lobe of the liver, the gallbladder may poorly attach to the liver or not attach at all, resulting in floating gallbladder or halting of gallbladder migration in the lesser omentum, mesocolon, abdominal wall/falciform ligament, retroduodenal area, and so on.

2. Failure of the gallbladder to migrate from the intrahepatic to extrahepatic surface at the 8th week of gestation may result in intrahepatic gallbladder.

3. The gallbladder may migrate to the left hepatic lobe rather than the right hepatic lobe, resulting in left-sided gallbladder.

4. If left umbilical vein atrophy and right umbilical vein persists, right left sided gallbladder will be formed. The persistent right umbilical vein may also be associated with atrophy or hypoplasia or agenesis of the right lobe of the liver with the consequence of retrohepatic or subdiaphragmatic gallbladder [1–3, 10–13].

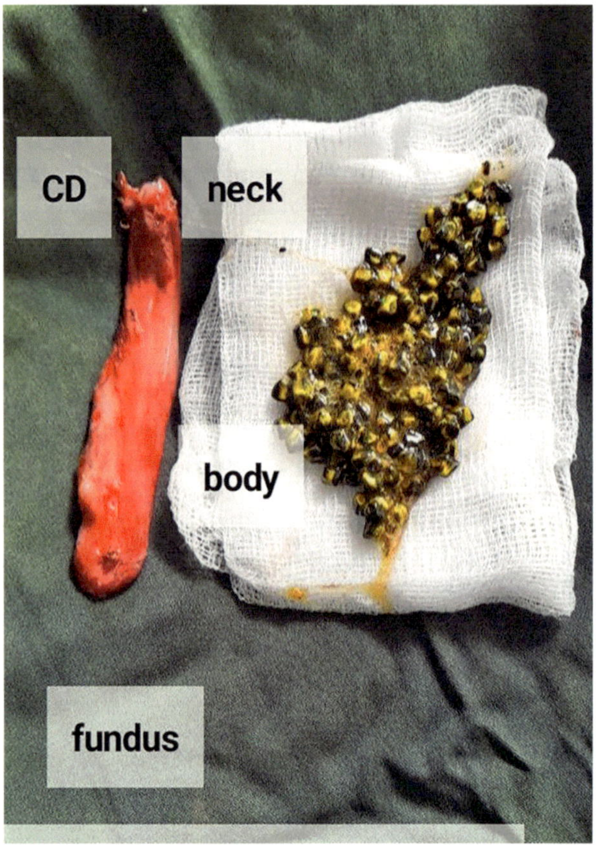

Figure 2.
Anatomical parts of gallbladder.

2.2 Gross anatomy of the gallbladder

The gallbladder is a pear-shaped organ located under the anterior inferior surface of the right lobe of the liver. It is adhered to the liver obliquely in the gallbladder fossa with the fundus extended anterolaterally and the neck extended inferomedially cranially and caudally, respectively. The gallbladder is 7–10-cm long, 3–4-cm wide, and 3-mm thick. Normally, it stores about 30–50 ml of bile, but it can accommodate up to 300 ml in its full distension. The anatomic parts of the gallbladder include the fundus, body, infundibulum, and neck. The fundus is the part of gallbladder that protrudes beyond the inferior surface of the liver. The part of the gallbladder between the fundus and infundibulum is the body. The tapering part from the body to the neck is the infundibulum. The neck connects the gallbladder with the hepatic duct through the cystic duct (**Figure 2**). Arterial supply is cystic artery from right hepatic artery. Cystic veins drain directly to portal veins. Lymphatic drainage is to the cystic lymph node at the gallbladder neck. Parasympathetic innervation is from the hepatic branch of the vagus nerve and sympathetic supply is from the hepatic and celiac plexus [13, 14].

2.3 Variants, epidemiology, and etiopathogenesis of gallbladder position anomalies

The gallbladder is normally located at the inferior surface of the liver between hepatic segments IV and V [1, 2, 15]. The gallbladder's fundus and body are covered by the peritoneum and adhered to the liver with loose connective tissue [1]. Any position or attachment other than this is defined as gallbladder malposition [1, 2, 13].

Gallbladder position anomalies are rarely occurring conditions, with an incidence of 0.1–0.7% [1, 6, 16]. More commonly occurring position anomalies as reported in the literature include floating gallbladder, left-sided gallbladder, intrahepatic gallbladder, and retro displaced gallbladders.

Relatively rarely occurring position anomalies include anterior abdominal wall, falciform ligament, mesocolon, lesser omentum, retrodoudenal, retrorenal, and retropancreatic gallbladders, among others [2, 8]. Some literature has concluded that left-sided gallbladder is the most common gallbladder position anomaly with an incidence of 0.1–0.7% based on a single-center retrospective review of gallbladder position anomalies found on laparoscopic cholecystectomy and the prevalence in patients evaluated by imaging [6, 17, 18]. However, Sreekanth et al. [13] performed dissection on 45 cadavers to determine incidence of floating gallbladder and reported an incidence of 4.4%. In addition, since the first reported case of left-sided gallbladder by Hochstetter [19] in 1886 and GBV by Wendel [20] in 1896, there have only been 150 and 500 cases of these conditions, respectively. Based on these figures, the most commonly occurring gallbladder malposition is floating gallbladder, which occurs in 5% of the population [5, 7, 13]. Left-sided gallbladder is the second most common anomaly, with an incidence of 0.1–1.2% [3, 4, 17]. The third most commonly occurring malposition is intrahepatic gallbladder [4, 11, 15]. Because sample sizes are small, these studies may not reflect true incidence. Hence, to determine true incidence, cadaver dissection or MRCP-based multicenter, prospective randomized clinical trials should be conducted.

2.3.1 Floating gallbladder

A floating gallbladder is a freely mobile gallbladder in the peritoneal cavity due to poor attachment of the gallbladder mesentery to the liver. Four subvariants of floating gallbladder are described in the literature [5, 7]. In type 1, there is no mesenteric attachment with the liver except at the gallbladder's cystic duct and artery. In type 2, there is mesenteric attachment between the gallbladder's body, fundus, and cystic duct with the liver, but the gallbladder is long, redundant, and tortuous. This allows for the gallbladder to wander around and it may end up in the pelvis, left upper quadrant, or anterior to the spine. In type 3, there is a freely mobile fundus, which may result in gallbladder fundus torsion. Types 1–3 are congenital conditions. In type 4, poor gallbladder mesenteric attachment may occur, as in cases of liver atrophy or cirrhosis, peritoneal fat loss secondary to aging, and weight loss [7, 13, 20, 21]. These abnormal attachments predispose the gallbladder to torsion, herniation, strangulation, and increased stone formation [22–39].

2.3.2 Left-sided gallbladder

Left-sided gallbladder is a rare malposition. It was first identified in 1886 by Hochstetter, and since then only 150 cases have been reported worldwide [3, 19]. The left-sided gallbladder is an anatomical variant in which the gallbladder is attached to the inferior surface of the left lobe of the liver to the left of the falciform ligament [10, 12, 14, 15, 40, 41]. Its prevalence is estimated to be 0.04–1.1% [3, 6, 22]. It is more common in females than males with a ratio of 2:1 [3] and the majority of cases are reported in Japan and Australia[]. According to current classification, there are three subtypes of left-sided gallbladder. Type 1 is called situs inversus viscerum. In this case, the gallbladder is found in the left upper quadrant of the liver. This condition is very rare. Type 2 is true left-sided gallbladder, also called sinistroposition. In this case, the gallbladder is found attached to the left lobe of the liver under hepatic segment III to the left of the falciform ligament. The exact etiology for this anomaly is not known, but there are three likely explanations. The first is the hypothesis that the gallbladder abnormally migrates from right to left. In this case, the cystic duct crosses the CBD to join at the right side. The second hypothesis is that an accessory gallbladder develops from the left duct and the main gallbladder either atrophies or fails to develop. In this case, the cystic duct joins the hepatic duct from the left side. In both cases, the cystic artery crosses the bile duct from right to left to supply the gallbladder. In true left-sided gallbladder, there is no associated intrahepatic vascular or duct anomalies. In the third hypothesis, the quadrate lobe of the liver fails to develop.

3. Right left-sided gallbladder is also called medio position or false left-sided gallbladder. In this case, the gallbladder is located normally, but the falciform ligament is abnormally located to the right of the gallbladder. During development, the right umbilical vein atrophies at the 6th week of gestation and the left umbilical vein is obliterated later and persists as the falciform ligament. If developmental disruption occurs to cause atrophy of the left umbilical vein and persistence of the right umbilical vein as the falciform ligament on the right side of the gallbladder, it falsely seems that the gallbladder is left sided [11, 22–24].

Associated anomalies with left-sided gallbladder include hepato-pancreatico-biliary (HPB) system, gastrointestinal system (GIS), and genitourinary system (GUS) anomalies. HPB anomalies occur more commonly than others and may include portal vein, bile duct, hepatic vein, and hepatic artery anomalies as well as hepatic segment IV atrophy and congenital hepatic cysts [3]. Portal vein anomalies include trifurcation, bifurcation, and other anomalies. Cystic duct anomalies in left-sided gallbladder may involve the cystic duct joining the right hepatic duct in 7.6% of cases, the left hepatic duct in 9.5% of cases, and the accessory duct in 2.4% of cases. The cystic duct joins the CBD from the right side in 65% of cases and from the left side in 9.5% of cases [42]. Other associated anomalies may include bile duct duplication, bile duct confluence in the umbilical fissure located to the left of the umbilical portion of the portal vein, and preduodenal portal vein, hepatic artery, and CBD anomalies. Annular pancreas, intestinal malrotation, and mobile right-sided colon are present [3]. Without considering situs inversus, 83% of left-sided gallbladder cases are true left-sided gallbladder and 16% are right left-sided gallbladder. The former has no associated vascular or biliary duct anomalies; rather, Calot's triangle is disrupted. The latter has associated vascular and duct anomalies. Almost all right left-sided gallbladders have portal vein and biliary duct anomalies, and 20% have hepatic vein anomalies [3, 6].

2.3.3 Intrahepatic gallbladder

An intrahepatic gallbladder is a completely or partially embedded gallbladder in hepatic parenchyma. In normal development, the gallbladder is expected to migrate from an intrahepatic to extrahepatic location during the 8th week of gestation. Failure of this migration results in intrahepatic gallbladder, which is considered as developmental position arrest. Its estimated incidence ranges between 0.1 and 0.7% [8, 10]. Though its etiology is not clearly known, developmental disruption of the differential growth of the hepatic bud is a possible cause of intrahepatic gallbladder. During development, the growth and differentiation of the hepatic bud is controlled by different transcription pathways. Any disruption in these pathways may result in position anomalies. If the caudal bud (pars cystica) grows beyond the cranial bud, the gallbladder may be buried in the hepatic parenchyma [8, 10, 13].

2.3.4 Retro position gallbladder

Types of retro position gallbladder include subhepatic, retrohepatic, and retroperitoneal gallbladder, all of which are rare conditions. Retrohepatic gallbladder is usually associated with marked atrophy of the right hepatic lobe or agenesis and anomalies of the right hepatic vein and portal vein [1, 4].

2.3.5 Mesocolic gallbladder

Mesocolic gallbladder is very rare. In one patient, Teke et al. [2] discovered the gallbladder embedded deeply within the proximal portion of the transverse mesocolon. Etiology is not clearly known, but it seems a gallbladder poorly attached to the free edge of the ventral mesentery during development results in failure of developmental gallbladder migration to the gallbladder fossa [2].

2.4 Clinical impacts of gallbladder position anomalies

The clinical significance of ectopic gallbladder may include the following:

- increased relative risk of cholelethiasis and its complications
- clinical confusion or misdiagnosis
- imaging misinterpretation
- increased associated biliary tree and vascular anomalies
- technical challenges during cholecystectomy

An ectopic gallbladder usually has poor function and a long narrow or curved cystic duct, which results in bile stasis and stone formation. Due to stasis, patients with ectopic gallbladder are more prone to develop complications like acute cholecystitis, gangrenous gallbladder, gallbladder empyema, perforation, peritonitis, and so on [1–7, 10]. Since there are no specific symptoms and signs for gallbladder malposition, it is usually diagnosed intraoperatively during laparoscopic cholecystectomy. Rarely, it may be diagnosed during preoperative evaluation for hepatic surgery. The prevalence of stones in an ectopic gallbladder may reach up to 60% [8, 10], which is higher than the 15–20% prevalence of stones in a normally located gallbladder. Most of these patients present with biliary colic or acute cholecystitis and its complications. Since the origin of nerves supply for ectopic gallbladder is not changed, these patients have similar clinical features with normal anatomical variants of gallbladder. They present with right upper abdomen pain that radiates to the shoulder and associated nausea, vomiting, and fever [3, 8]. Sometimes some gallbladder ectopia may pose clinical confusion. For example, retroperitoneal or retrohepatic gallbladders with acute cholecystitis may have costovertebral angle tenderness instead of typical right abdominal pain, which leads to misdiagnosis of gallbladder ectopia as acute pyelonephritis [1, 2]. Delayed diagnosis and intervention may result in retroperitoneal gallbladder perforation with accumulation of bile or abscess, which may be misinterpreted as perinephric abscess during imaging [1].

The clinical sequelae of floating gallbladder includes GBV, gallbladder herniation, and gallbladder strangulation by the tip of the omentum.

GBV is a rare clinical condition; only about 500 cases have been reported since the first case reported by Wendel in 1896 [20]. Its incidence is estimated to be 1 in 365,520 hospital admissions [7, 21]. It is more common in females than males with a 3:1 ratio [7, 21, 22]. GBV is defined as twisting of the gallbladder with mesentery along its longitudinal axis [7, 20–22]. Its etiology is not known, but anomalous gallbladder mesentery attachment with liver seems to be a predisposing factor [7, 21, 22].

Additional predisposing factors include old age, weight loss, cirrhosis, kyphosis, vigorous adjacent gastrointestinal peristalsis, cystic artery atherosclerosis, and abnormally high insertion of cystic duct. Even though GBV can occur at any age, it usually occurs in those aged between 60 and 80 years [7, 22, 33–39]. This is due to increased loss of mesenteric fat and tissue elasticity in the elderly, which results in a freely mobile gallbladder. Kyphosis will increase the anteroposterior diameter of the abdomen, conferring adequate space for a wandering gallbladder to be twisted. The direction of torsion could be clockwise or counterclockwise; both occur with equal frequency. The direction of the twist is likely determined by the origin of vigorous peristalsis. Gastric and transverse colon peristalsis result in clockwise and counterclockwise directions, respectively. Based on degree of rotation, GBV can be classified as either complete (>180 degrees) or incomplete (<180 degrees) [7, 21, 33–39]. This classification has clinical importance. The former presents with acute onset of symptoms and short duration, whereas the latter present presents with intermittent symptoms of relatively long duration [7, 21, 22].

Because they are both rare and share similar clinical presentations, GBV is often misdiagnosed as calculous acute cholecystitis. Nowadays, about 75% of GBV cases are diagnosed intraoperatively. Late diagnosis and surgical intervention are associated with an increased mortality rate of 6% and thus preoperative diagnosis is recommended to decrease mortality and morbidity [7, 33–39].

2.4.1 Gallbladder herniation

Wandering gallbladder may herniate into foramen of Winslow (lesser sac). For example, in one review of six cases [23], floating gallbladder herniated into the lesser sac; half of patients had hernia with GBV and half did not have GBV. Kim et al. [5] reviewed fourteen cases and reported only four cases of gallbladder herniation with GBV; the remaining ten cases had gallbladder herniation with acute cholecystitis. Floating gallbladder may herniate into anterior abdominal wall defects [25, 27–32], most commonly parastomal gallbladder herniation [29]. Unusual gallbladder herniations are also reported in the literature. For example, [31] reported a case of Spigelian gallbladder hernia, [27] reported a case of inguinal gallbladder hernia, and [28] reported a case of femoral gallbladder hernia. Another possible gallbladder hernia is to the thorax [32]. Almost all gallbladder hernias are diagnosed intraoperatively. Floating gallbladder may also be strangulated by the tip of the omentum, which is attached to the anterior abdominal wall [25]. Female gender and old age are sole risk factors. The complications of gallbladder herniation include gallbladder torsion, cholecystitis, Mirizzi syndrome, incarceration, and ischemia [27–32, 43].

Intrahepatic gallbladder may mimic liver or cystic masses during diagnostic imaging, which results in extended investigation and delay in diagnosis. This delay may cause intrahepatic gallbladder perforation and liver abscess that may be considered as a hydatid cyst during imaging [8, 10, 44, 45]. Laparoscopic cholecystectomy in intrahepatic gallbladder is challenging because it requires hepatotomy. Intrahepatic gallbladder should be diagnosed in the preoperative period before any hepatic surgery. Failure to do so may result in gallbladder and biliary tree injury with postoperative bile leak [44, 45].

Gallbladder position anomalies pose technical challenges during standard laparoscopic cholecystectomy. Malposition changes the normal position of Calot's triangle, which changes the normal relationship of the gallbladder and biliary tree. Thus, safe dissection techniques are not practical here without modifications. Patients with gallbladder malposition also have increased rates of associated biliary tree and vascular anomalies. Due to both technical challenges and associated anomalies, laparoscopic cholecystectomy is associated with high rates of bile duct injury, ranging from 4.4 to 7.3%; in normally located gallbladders, the rate of bile duct injury is 0.7% [44–48].

2.5 Diagnosis and management

Most patients with gallbladder malposition are diagnosed intraoperatively during surgery for symptomatic cholelithiasis and its complications or HPB surgery. Preoperative diagnosis will help in planning and delivering safe surgical treatment. This is not possible during management of patients with biliary colic or its complications because initial imaging modalities like ultrasound (US) are enough to give treatment. However, US is not good at detecting ectopic gallbladder; its positive predictive value is only 2.7% [18]. So, surgeons should have sound knowledge of anatomical variants of the gallbladder and biliary tree. Its intraoperative identification is the mainstay of prevention of complications. The gold standard investigation modality for gallbladder malposition is MRCP [18, 47, 48], thus all patients scheduled for hepatic surgery should be evaluated for gallbladder position anomalies and associated biliary duct, vascular, and other anomalies using MRCP.

2.5.1 Left-sided gallbladder

Patients with left-sided gallbladder usually present with biliary colic or acute cholecystitis, and diagnosis is made intraoperatively. Typically, patients undergo preoperative US that detects gallbladder stones but fails to detect the position anomaly. Whenever cystic lesion are found in an atypical location and the gallbladder is not found in its normal location, the possibility of ectopic gallbladder should be considered and computed tomography (CT) or MRCP evaluation should be performed [18, 26, 40–42]. CT will show the gallbladder located to the left of the round ligament with a positive predictive value of 60% [18]. MRCP will detect the position anomaly and associated biliary duct anomalies. Associated vascular anomalies require CT angiography.

2.5.2 Gallbladder volvulus

Nowadays only 26% of gallbladder torsions are diagnosed preoperatively [7, 21]. This is because of their rare prevalence and similar clinical presentation to a common gallbladder pathology, acute cholecystitis. Similarly, there are no specific radiology features during initial imaging.

Ultrasound. Multidetector computed tomography (MDCT) and magnetic resonance imaging (MRI) have better sensitivity and specificity, but are not cost effective in emergency situations. A high level of suspicion is important to diagnose these patients early. The typical patient with gallbladder torsion is a cachectic and kyphotic elderly woman, aged 60–80 years, presenting with right upper abdomen pain, nausea, and vomiting. On examination, vital signs are stable, and the patient is nonestrous and nontoxic with a globular mass in the right upper abdomen [7, 21–23, 33, 43]. Laboratory studies will show leukocytosis and elevated c-reactive protein (CRP). Even though they are usually missed, there are features on US, including an enlarged and distended gallbladder with increased wall thickness, absent stones and pericholecystic fluid collection, gallbladder displacement down and away from the liver and lying in a transverse position, cone-shaped hyperechoic lesion to the right side of gallbladder neck (i.e., twisted cystic duct) (**Figure 3**). These clinical and US findings are suggestive of gallbladder torsion. Nonenhanced CT scan has similar findings to US. GBV diagnosis can be confirmed with MDCT or MRCP. MDCT findings show an enlarged and distended gallbladder, fluids between the liver and gallbladder, and an intra-gallbladder hyperdense lesion with crease (**Figure 4**). MRCP shows a distended gallbladder, tapering cystic duct, and V-shaped distortion of extrahepatic ducts [22, 37–39]. Despite all these investigation modalities, the majority of patients are still diagnosed intraoperatively. Intraoperative findings are black gallbladder with inflamed surrounding peritoneum and hugely distended gallbladder in transverse position and a twisted cystic duct (**Figure 5**). Management involves aspiration and derotation of the gallbladder followed by cholecystectomy. Histopathological study shows hemorrhagic necrosis. The gold standard for surgical management is laparoscopic cholecystectomy [6, 14, 15, 40, 42]. However, in the absence of expertise and

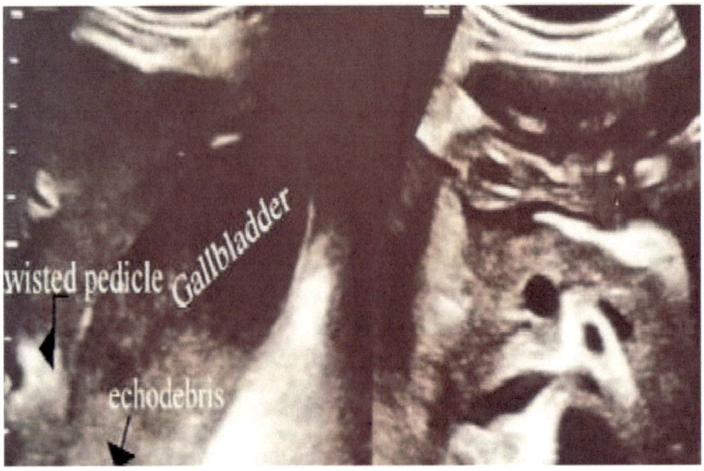

Figure 3.
US of GBV patient showing distended GB in transverse lye, twisted CD & pericholecystic fluid. (Taken from Musefa Redwan Abdella and Amsalu Midaso Titole) [21].

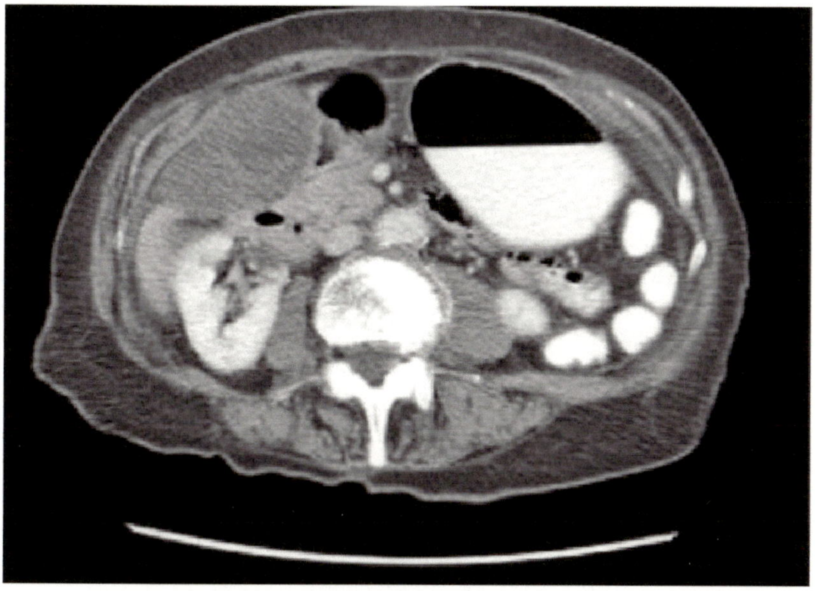

Figure 4.
CT of GBV distended GB without stones. (Taken from Bhama) [33].

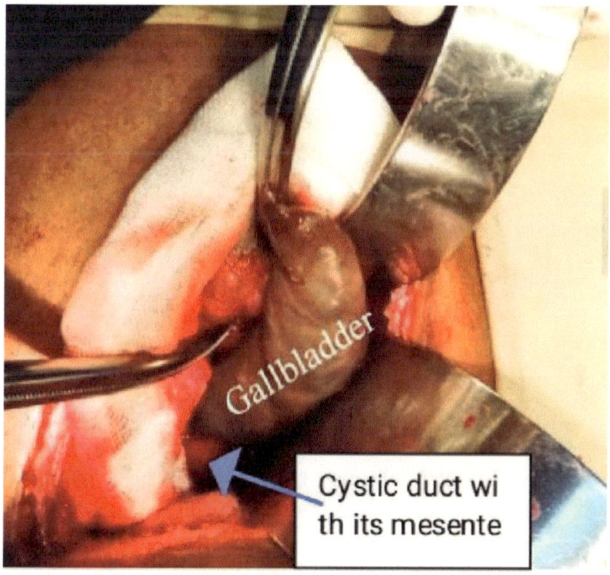

Figure 5.
Intraoperative clockwise twisted GB. (Taken from Musefa Redwan Abdella and Amsalu Midaso Titole) [21].

setup and in the presence of absolute contraindication for laparoscopic cholecystectomy, open cholecystectomy is an option.

2.5.3 Intrahepatic gallbladder

These patients usually present with symptomatic cholelethiasis and its complications. Stones and intrahepatic malposition can be diagnosed with US. CT may be needed when cystic liver mass lesions are considered in the differential diagnosis. MRCP should be considered to assess associated biliary duct and vascular anomalies.

Management is laparoscopic cholecystectomy after hepatotomy. To avoid bile duct injuries, the cystic duct must be identified at the cystic plate and followed to the gallbladder. In case of difficulties due to poor exposure and bleeding, conversion to open surgery is recommended [8, 10]. The approach to open surgery is right subcostal incision with extension to the thorax [44]. Cholecystectomy should be done in cases of incidental finding of ectopic gallbladder to avoid future clinical and imaging confusion [1, 2]. The most important thing in managing symptomatic ectopic gallbladder patients is to prevent bile duct injuries. To perform and deliver safe surgical treatment, the following measures are recommended:

1. Preoperative diagnosis of gallbladder malposition and associated anomalies. This will help to plan the appropriate surgical approach to complete the surgery safely.

2. Technical modification of laparoscopic cholecystectomy. This may include port modification, such as adding port sites [40, 45] or shifting port sites (e.g., [15]). Patient position modifications can also be considered (e.g., [40]) to identify left-sided gallbladder. The patient should be put in the supine position first and then moved to the lithotomy position. Dissection technique modifications like falciform ligament lifting and fundus first approach are highly recommended [15, 40].

3. Conversion cholecystectomy. Surgeons should not hesitate to convert to open cholecystectomy whenever there is difficulty or doubtful anatomy.

4. Fundus first cholecystectomy

5. Routine intraoperative cholangiography, which will show detailed biliary anatomy. This is the key to performing safe surgery.

6. Surgeons should have detailed knowledge of the gallbladder and biliary tree and vascular anatomical variants. This is important to decrease mortality and morbidity.

Gallbladder malposition patients may present with severe calculus cholecystitis or calculus cholecystitis due to stasis like gallbladder empyema or retroperitoneal or hepatic abscess. These patients may be considered high risk for surgery. In these cases, percutaneous drainage with appropriate antibiotics and interval laparoscopic cholecystectomy is recommended [45].

Retroperitoneal and retrohepatic gallbladder patients may present with right costovertebral angle tenderness that can be confused with hepatic mass lesions or cysts as well as renal cysts or masses on preoperative US and CT scan. MRCP is the gold standard diagnostic modality in these patients.

Dissection and resection of these deep-seated gallbladders is technically difficult [1]. Laparoscopic cholecystectomy can be considered, but the team should prepared for conversion cholecystectomy.

US and CT do not usually detect anatomical anomalies, though they can identify gallbladder stones. If the gallbladder is adjacent to the transverse colon on CT scan, MRCP should be considered to confirm diagnosis of mesocolic gallbladder. Laparoscopic cholecystectomy with technical modification is a safe procedure, but surgeons should always keep in mind the possibility of conversion to open cholecystectomy [6, 15, 16, 40, 42].

3. Conclusion

Gallbladder positions anomalies are rarely occurring conditions in clinical practice. Though further study is needed, the most commonly occurring variants in descending order of frequency are floating gallbladder, left-sided gallbladder, intrahepatic gallbladder, and retro placed gallbladder. Ectopic gallbladders are prone to increased stone formation and related complications due to the impaired function of the gallbladder. Most position anomalies are diagnosed intraoperatively during surgery for cholelithiasis or its complications because of their rare prevalence and lack of specific clinical and imaging features. Despite advancement in radiological technology, preoperative diagnosis remains difficult; the preoperative diagnosis rate is about 20%. Gallbladder position anomalies have clinical sequelae like GBV, gallbladder herniation with strangulation in floating gallbladder, and gallbladder perforation with liver abscess in intrahepatic gallbladder. Gallbladder malposition is usually associated with biliary tree and vascular anomalies that together with changed anatomy predispose patients to increased rates of bile duct injuries (7.3%).

To prevent these devastating complications, anomalies must be diagnosed preoperatively, especially in patients scheduled for hepatic resection or liver transplantation. The surgeon should have detailed knowledge of anatomical variants of the biliary system and should always consider their possible prescience during laparoscopic cholecystectomy. When position anomalies are discovered suddenly during a procedure, technical modifications to the procedure are mandatory. These may include port site or patient position modifications, falciform ligament lifting, or fundus first approach when needed. Routine intraoperative cholangiography in laparoscopic cholecystectomy and intraoperative liver US to view biliary duct and vascular structures in hepatic surgery decreases the rate of bile duct and vascular injuries.

Acknowledgements

I would like to thank IntechOpen for providing an Open Access Publishing Fee support since I and my institution could not afford the funding of publishing the manuscript in Open Access.

Conflict of interest

Author declares none.

Acronyms and abbreviations

GBPAs	gallbladder position anomalies
GBV	gallbladder volvulus
GBH	gallbladder herniation
FGB	floating gallbladder
LtSGB	left-sided gallbladder
RLtSGB	right left-sided gallbladder
IHGB	intrahepatic gallbladder
HPB	hepato-pancreatico-biliary system

Author details

Musefa Redwan
Yirgalem Hospital Medical Collage and Yirgalem General Hospital, Yirgalem, Ethiopia

*Address all correspondence to: musefaredwan8@gmail.com

References

[1] David E, Charles A, Stanleyr M. Gallbladder ectopia: A review of anomalies of position. 1974;**121**(2): 396-400. DOI: 10.2214/ajr.121.2.396

[2] Teke Z, Akcam AT. Complete mesocolic malposition of the gallbladder: An unusual case report with literature's review. Ulusal Travma ve Acil Cerrahi Dergisi. 2022;**28**:557-561

[3] Lee H et al. Anatomic variation of patient with a left-sided gallbladder. The Annals of Surgical Treatment and Research. 2019;**97**(6):302-308

[4] Gu W, Tong Z. Ectopic gallbladder: A case report and review of the literature. Asian Journal of Surgery. July 2020;**43**(9):1-3. December 2029. DOI: 10.1016/j.asjsur.2020.05.017

[5] Kim WS et al. Strangulated gallbladder by the lesser Omentum. Soonchunhyang Medical Science. Dec 2020;**26**(2):9194

[6] Strong RW et al. Surgical implications of left sided gallbladder. The American Journal of Surgery. July 2013;**206**(1): 59-63. DOI: 101016/jamjsurg201210035

[7] Boer J, Boerma D, de Vries Reilingh TS. A gallbladder torsion presenting as acute cholecystitis in an elderly woman: A case report. Journal of Medical Case Reports. Cholecystitis in an intrahepatic gallbladder, international journal of surgery. September 2017;**4**(9):3177-3179. DOI: 10.1186/1752-1947-5-588

[8] Chandrasekar G, Nagappa V. Cholelithiasis in an intrahepatic gallbladder. International Journal of Surgery. 2017;**4**(9):3177-3379

[9] Sahu SYVM, Yang SNAA. Cell sources for treating diabetes [internet]. In: Stem Cells in Clinic and Research. London, UK: InTech; 2011:156-163. DOI: 10.5772/24174

[10] Muguti G, Muchuweti D, Munyika AA. Congenital duplex gallbladder anomaly presenting as gangrenous perforated intrahepatic cholecystitis A case report and review of literature. East and Central African Journal of Surgery. 2013;**18**(2)

[11] Banchini F, Capelli P. Left sided gallbladder clinical and anatomical implication. Anatomy & Embryology of Biliary Tract. Surgical Clinics of North America. 2014;**94**:203-217. DOI: 10.5772/intechopen.92000

[12] Keplinger, Bloomston. Anatomy and embryology of the biliary tract. Surgical Clinics. 2014;**94**:203217. DOI: 10.1016/j.suc.2014.01.001surgical.theclinics.com.00396109/14/$

[13] Sreekanth T. Incidence of floating/wandering gall bladders: A cadaveric study and its clinical implications. International Journal of Anatomy and Research. 2017;**5**(1):3338-3341. DOI: 10.16965/L.2016.470

[14] Qureshi. Aberrant presentation of the gallbladder during laparoscopic cholecystectomy. JSLS: Journal of the Society of Laparoendoscopic Surgeons. 2009;**13**:605-607

[15] Nastosetal C. Methods of safe laparoscopic cholecystectomy for left-sided (sinistroposition) gallbladder: A report of two cases and a review of safe techniques. International Journal of Surgery Case Reports. 2014;**5**:769-773

[16] Idu M, Jakimowicz J, Iuppa A, Cuschieri A. Hepatobiliary anatomy in patients with transposition of the

gallbladder: Implications for safe laparoscopic cholecystectomy. British Journal of Surgery. 1996;**83**:14421443

[17] Yadav A, Jain NB, Ray S, Nundy S. The ectopic gall bladder: A review. International Journal of Health Sciences. 2022;**6**(S6):32473253. DOI: 10.53730/ijhs.v6nS6.10054

[18] Hsu SL, Chen TY, Huang TL, Sun CK, Concejero AM, Tsang LL, et al. Left sided gallbladder: Its clinical significance and imaging presentations. World Journal of Gastroenterology. 2007;**13**:6404-6409. DOI: 10.3748/wjg.v13.i47.6404

[19] Hochstetter F. Anomaliemder Pfortaderunddernabelvenein verbindungmitdefectoder Linkscage dergallenblase. Archivfür Mikroskopische Anatomieund Entwicklungsmechanik. 1886;**3**:369-384

[20] Wendel AV. VI. A case of floating gallbladder and kidney complicated by cholelethiasis, with per- foration of the gallbladder. Annals of Surgery. 1898;**27**(2):199-202

[21] Abdella MR, Titole AM. The clinical case report of gallbladder volvulus. Enormous Journal of Medical Sciences and Current Research. 2022;**2**(3):1040, 1-6. DOI: 10.56558/journal.ejmscr.1001040

[22] Pu TW et al. Acute body-neck torsion of the gallbladder. WJG. 2014;**20**(38):1-3

[23] Nguyen TH, Tran KH, Le XA, Nguyen HV, Ha QV. Gallbladder volvulus and hernia through the foramen of Winslow: A case report. Journal of Surgical Case Reports. 2020;**93**(10):rjaa424. DOI: 10.1093/jscr/rjaa424

[24] Ben Ismail I et al. Cholecystitis in a midline gallbladder: A rare ectopic location. International Journal of Surgery Case Reports. 2022;**93**:106969I

[25] Kohgaetal A. Strangulatedp gallbladder caused by a tip of the omentum attached to the abdominal wall: A case report. Journal of Surgical Case Reports. 2017;**7**:1-3

[26] Gelevski R et al. True left sided gallbladder (TLSG) as incidental finding on laparoscopic cholecystectomy: Case report. JMS. 2021;**4**(1):50-53. UDC:616.366-089.81

[27] Tajti J, Pieler J, Ábrahám S, et al. Incarcerated gallbladder in inguinal hernia: A case report and literature review. BMC Gastroenterology. 2020;**20**:425. DOI: 10.1186/s12876-020-01569-5

[28] LK, De Jesus RB, Torri GB, Momo M, Rodrgues LK, Ameida Ghezzi CL, et al. Gallbladder protrusion through the groin region—a very unusual femora hernia. BJR|Case Reports. 2019;**5**:20180035

[29] Rogers et al. Gallbladder complicating a parastomal hernia. Journal of Surgical Case Reports. 2019;**4**:1-3. DOI: 10.1093/jscr/rjz107

[30] Kumari S. Case report and operative management of obstructed epigastric hernia containing gall bladder: a rare entity. International Journal of Surgery. 2020;7:3805-3807

[31] KM, SHX C, Ying F, AKH C. Gallbladder herniation through ventral hernia: A case report. Open Journal of Clinical and Medical Case Reports. 2019;(4):rjz2017

[32] Ennis G, Venade G, Silva Marques J, Batista P, Abreu Nunes A, Constantino J, et al. Intrathoracic acute cholecystitis. European Journal of Case Reports in Internal Medicine. 2020;**7**(11):3805-3807. DOI: 10.12890/2020001764

[33] Bhama AR. The diagnostic dilemma of gallbladder volvulus report of a case.

General Internal Medicine and Clinical Innovations. 2016, 2015;**1**(2):26-29. DOI: 10.15761/GIMCI.1000108

[34] Croce, Licata. Gallbladder volvulus: A case report. Journal of Medical Case Reports. 2021;**15**:494. DOI: 10.1186/s13256021031157

[35] Reddy K et al. Laparoscopic derotation and cholecystectomy of torsion gallbladder. JSLS: Journal of the Society of Laparoendoscopic Surgeons. 2005;**9**:238-240

[36] Setty N, RS et al. Cadaveric floating gallbladder and its clinical significance a case report. International Journal of Current Research and Review. 2013;**15**(1):494

[37] Miyata T, Sannomiya Y, Nagayama T, et al. Preoperative diagnosis of gallbladder torsion by magnetic resonance cholangiopancreatography: A case report. Clinical Case Reports. 2022;**10**:e05487. DOI: 10.1002/ccr3.5487

[38] Daniel, George K, Dhan T. Torsion of the gallbladder: A systematic review. HPB: The Official Journal of the International Hepato Pancreato Biliary Association. 2012;**14**:669-672. DOI: 10.1111/j.14772574.2012.00513.x

[39] Usui M, Matsuda S, Suzuki H, Ogura Y. Preoperative diagnosis of gallbladder torsion by magnetic resonance cholangio pancreatography. Scandinavian Journal of Gastroenterology. 2000;**35**:218-222

[40] Reddy PK, Subramanian RV, Yuvaraja S. Laparoscopic cholecystectomy for left-sided gallbladder (sinistroposition). JSLS: Journal of the Society of Laparoendoscopic Surgeons. 2005;**9**(3):356-357

[41] Maetani Y, Itoh K, Kojima N, Tabuchi T, Shibata T, Asonuma K, et al. Portal vein anomaly associated with deviation of the ligamentum teres to the right and malposition of the gallbladder. Radiology. 1998;**207**:723-728

[42] Pereira R, Perera M, Roberts M, Avramovic J. Surgical approach to a left-sided gallbladder. BML Case Reports. 2019;**12**(8):e230681. DOI: 10.1136/bcr-2019-230681

[43] Paolino LA, Millan M, Bossi M, Champault G, Barrat C. Herniation of the gallbladder within a hernia of the abdominal wall associated with Mirizzi syndrome. JSCR. 2011;**4**:3

[44] Audi P, Noronha F, Rodrigues J. Intrahepatic gallbladder - A case report and review of literature. The internet. Journal of Surgery. 2009;**14**(1):6, 1-4

[45] Donati et al. Antitypical presentation of intrahepatic perforated cholecystitis: a modern indication to open cholecystectomy. Report of a case. BMC Surgery. 2014;**14**:6

[46] Kocabiyik. Abnormal localization of gallbladder and atresia of superior part of duodenum. SDÜ Tıp Fakültesi Dergisi. 2008;**15**(1):38-41

[47] Mattone E et al. Dystopic gallbladder: Rendez vousand fluorescence. Clinical Case Reports. 2018;**6**(3):522526b. DOI: 101002/ccr31130

[48] Tarakj A, Kocabiyik et al. Successful surgical Management of Unusual Gallbladder Anatomy through Laparoscopic Cholecystectomy of ectopic gallbladder. Cures. 2021;**13**(11):e19884. DOI: 107759/cureus1988

Chapter 3

EUS of the Gallbladder

Landon Kozai and Larissa Fujii-Lau

Abstract

Endoscopic ultrasound (EUS) is an increasingly used imaging modality in the diagnosis and management of biliary disease. The advantage of EUS is that it allows for a precise examination of the pancreaticobiliary system due to the proximity of the endoscopic probe within the gastrointestinal tract. As EUS becomes more prevalent within gastroenterology practice, clinicians should become familiar with the endosonographic findings of the gallbladder. This chapter will review normal endosonographic gallbladder anatomy in addition to benign and malignant gallbladder pathology. The identifying endosonographic characteristics of gallbladder lesions will be discussed. We will also provide a brief review of EUS-guided tissue acquisition of the gallbladder.

Keywords: endoscopic ultrasound, EUS, gallbladder, biliary, fine needle aspiration, fine needle biopsy

1. Introduction

Endoscopic ultrasound (EUS) has become an important tool in the diagnosis and management of gallbladder disease. EUS utilizes high ultrasound frequencies of 5 mHz to 20 mHz and produces images with high spatial resolution, allowing for a more precise evaluation than with transabdominal ultrasound (TAUS) [1, 2]. Gallbladder structures can be closely examined for fine details such as depth of tumor invasion or subtle morphologic features of small gallbladder lesions which are normally obscured to examiners using TAUS. It also offers a unique advantage over TAUS by allowing the operator to perform fine needle aspiration (FNA) or fine needle biopsy (FNB) for tissue sampling at a closer location to the gallbladder. EUS is often preceded by cross-sectional imaging such as computed tomography (CT) or magnetic resonance cholangiopancreatography (MRCP) due to the unpredictable orientation of the gallbladder that is difficult to predict with EUS alone [3].

EUS of the gallbladder itself is often overlooked during the EUS examination. Endosonographers should be competent in recognizing normal and pathologic findings of the gallbladder and biliary tree. This chapter will provide an overview of the normal anatomy of the biliary tree as well as typical endosonographic characteristics of both benign and malignant gallbladder pathology. With the increasing use of EUS in clinical practice, it is important for physicians to be proficient in the interpretation of EUS findings and to be able to integrate these findings into the overall management of patients with gallbladder disease.

2. Normal gallbladder anatomy

The gallbladder is a pear-shaped organ in the right upper quadrant of the abdomen. It is located within a fossa separating the right and quadrate lobes on the liver [4]. The fundus of the gallbladder is the widest and most distal aspect, which tapers into the body, followed by the neck (or infundibulum) at its most proximal aspect. The neck lies in the porta hepatis and is connected to the cystic duct, forming a hook-like shape, which then drains into the common bile duct in a downward fashion. Within the cystic ducts are valvular structures known as the valves of Heister, which contribute to the controlled release of bile from the gallbladder. The fundus of the gallbladder abuts the anterior abdominal wall due to its projection beyond the inferior border of the liver. In some people, there is a benign outpouching of the fundus known as a Phrygian cap. A pouch-like structure located near the infundibulum may also be present and is known as Hartmann's pouch [5].

EUS of the gallbladder can be performed from 3 major areas: the gastroesophageal junction/fundus of the stomach, antrum/duodenal bulb, and descending duodenum. The endosonographer should become familiar with varying positions required to obtain adequate views of the gallbladder and its surrounding structures in each of these areas. EUS probe positioning and maneuvers to obtain adequate views of the surrounding gallbladder structures, and their unique orientations at each viewpoint are beyond the scope of this chapter. Notable structures observed from these positions in addition to the gallbladder itself include the portal vein, hepatic artery, right and left hepatic ducts, common hepatic duct, common bile duct, cystic duct, and inferior vena cava [5].

The layers of the gallbladder wall consist of the surface epithelium, lamina propria, muscularis propria, perimuscular subserosal connective tissue, and serosa [6]. On EUS, the normal gallbladder wall is depicted by three distinct layers. The innermost hyperechoic layer represents a boundary echo [3]. The middle layer is hypoechoic and consists of the mucosa, the muscularis propria, and the fibrous layer of the subserosa. The outer layer is hyperechoic, consisting of the adipose portion of the subserosal layer and serosa (**Figure 1**) [7–9]. A normal gallbladder wall is less than 4 mm in thickness. The inner layer of the gallbladder should demonstrate a smooth contour [10].

3. Abnormal gallbladder findings

The differential diagnosis of abnormal gallbladder lesions on EUS can be broadly divided into protuberant and wall-thickening lesions [10]. Protuberant lesions describe anomalies confined to the luminal surface of the gallbladder wall. Features such as lesion size, pedunculation, morphology, surface characteristics, and internal echo are considered in formulating the differential diagnosis.

Gallbladder wall thickening refers to lesions that cause the gallbladder wall to become diffusely thickened with a diameter $\geq$ 4 mm. Features such as the extent of wall thickening, surface structure, disruption of the gallbladder wall layers and presence of Rokitansky-Aschoff sinuses are considered in the differential diagnosis.

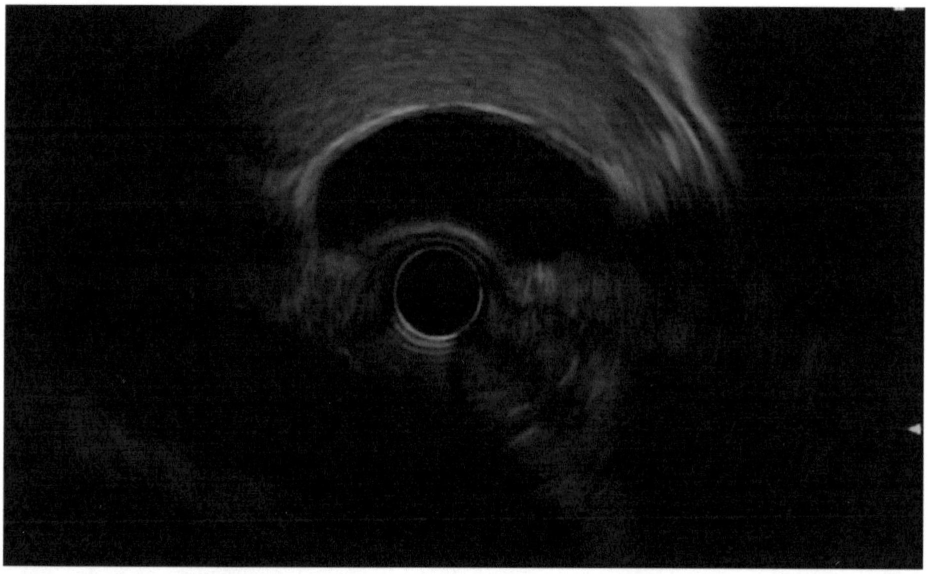

Figure 1.
Normal EUS of the gallbladder demonstrating multiple wall layers.

4. Protuberant lesions

Protuberant gallbladder lesions can be divided by morphologic features into pedunculated and sessile lesions. The differential diagnosis of protuberant and sessile lesions is important in the assessment of a lesion's malignant potential. Pedunculated lesions may include gallbladder polyps, adenomas, and gallbladder carcinoma, while sessile lesions may signify gallbladder carcinoma, adenomyosis, and sludge. While sessile shape is strongly associated with gallbladder carcinoma, pedunculated shape is more likely to represent a benign lesion or an early stage carcinoma confined to the mucosa [11].

Another way to further classify protuberant lesions is to subdivide them into neoplastic and non-neoplastic lesions. Neoplastic lesions are either adenomatous or carcinomatous, and non-neoplastic lesions largely consist of gallbladder polyps, and can be described as focal elevations or protrusions easily distinguished from the surrounding mucosa (**Figure 2**) [12]. The majority of gallbladder polyps are asymptomatic and may be discovered incidentally. Size of the lesion is also important; protuberant lesions greater than 20 mm in diameter are often easy to detect, even by TAUS, and are often malignant in nature. However, for those less than 20 mm, the differential diagnosis is broad, and they are challenging to diagnose by EUS features alone. Therefore, knowledge of the specific endosonographic features unique to each etiology, both benign and malignant is essential.

4.1 Benign protuberant gallbladder lesions

4.1.1 Gallbladder polyps

EUS is not ideal at distinguishing different types of gallbladder polyps. Cholesterol polyps are the most common type of gallbladder polyps, and account for approximately

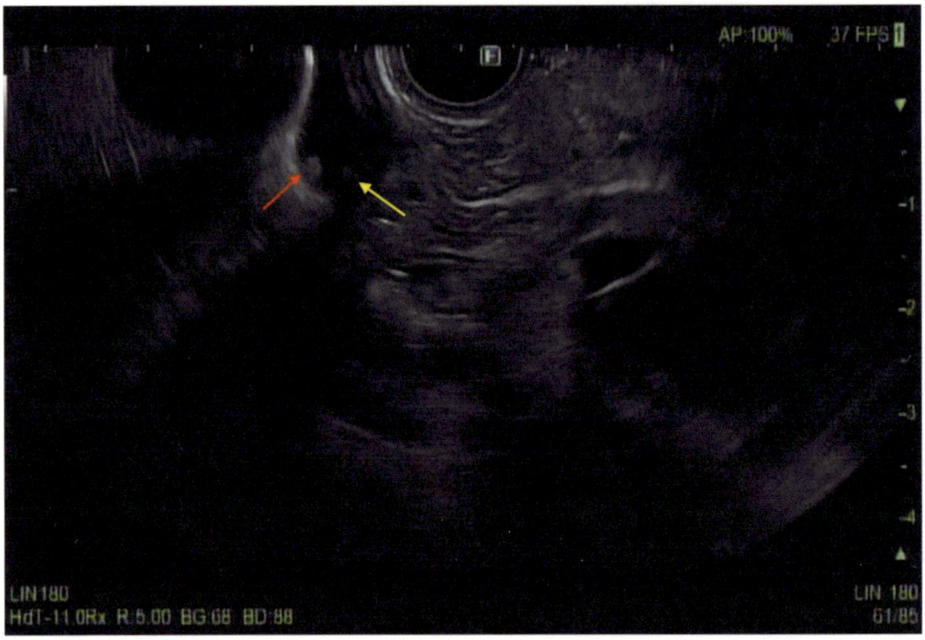

Figure 2.
Gallbladder polyp (red arrow) depicted next to a gallstone (yellow arrow).

95% of all raised gallbladder lesions [3]. Gallbladder polyps ≤10 mm are likely to be cholesterol polyps, but malignant polyps of this size are also found on occasion. Cholesterol polyps are pedunculated lesions, typically round in shape with a notched granular surface, and have a hyperechoic to isoechoic internal echo with echogenic punctiform foci representing cholesterosis [1, 10]. Larger cholesterol polyps greater than 10 mm in diameter may be more irregular or oblong in shape [1]. As cholesterol polyps enlarge to a size greater than 10 mm, they become more lobulated in appearance, and the internal echo decreases, taking on an appearance that can appear similar to adenomas or gallbladder cancer [10]. Due to this, they may be difficult to distinguish from malignant polyps and therefore cholecystectomy may be considered in this setting. Contrast-enhanced US may be useful for differentiating benign polyps from cancer [13].

The other types of gallbladder polyps are much less common. Hyperplastic polyps are benign protrusions consisting of hyperplasia of the gallbladder mucosa. They are typically ≥10 mm in diameter with a smooth surface, papillated or lobulated morphology, pedunculated base, and have uniform low echogenicity [12]. Inflammatory polyps are typically a result of chronic inflammation. They represent focal epithelial proliferations of inflammatory cells and are often associated with chronic cholecystitis. They consist of granulation and fibrous tissue and have no malignant potential. They are typically <10 mm in size and are often associated with chronic cholecystitis [14, 15]. On ultrasound, they may appear sessile or pedunculated. The internal echo is homogeneous and more echogenic than the liver parenchyma [15].

4.1.2 Cholelithiasis and sludge

Gallstones appear on EUS as intraluminal hyperechoic foci with or without acoustic shadowing (**Figure 2**) [16]. They may be gravity dependent. One study of

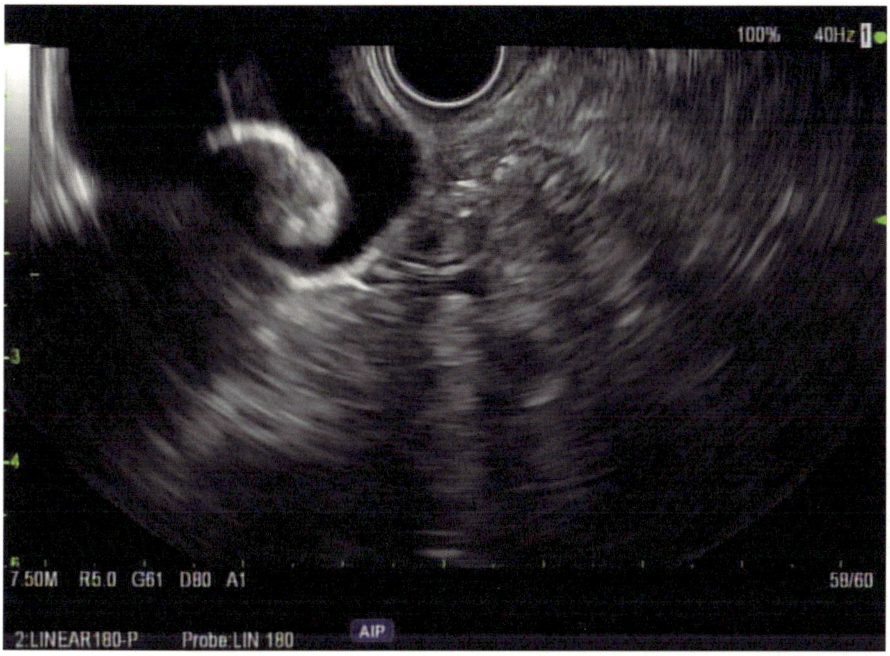

Figure 3.
Hyperechoic gallstone with shadowing.

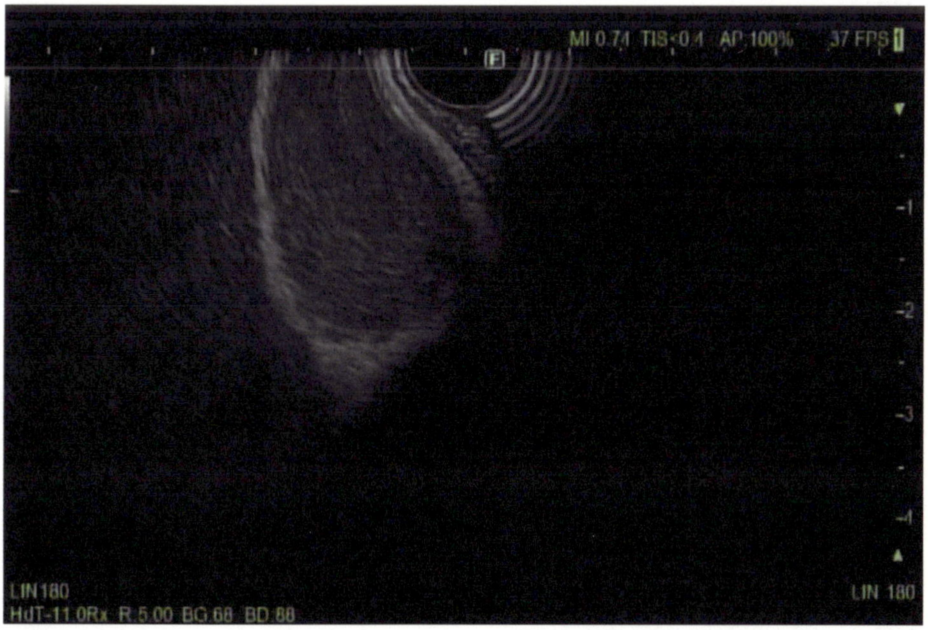

Figure 4.
Biliary sludge.

patients presenting with typical biliary pain and a negative initial TAUS found that small, undetected culprit gallstones less than or equal to 3 mm in size were often found in the infundibulum or cystic duct when examined by EUS [16]. EUS is also useful for the detection of biliary sludge or microlithiasis in patients presenting with seemingly idiopathic acute pancreatitis (IAP). The sensitivity of EUS for detecting a case in IAP surpasses that of MRCP [17–21]. Biliary sludge appears as a gravity-dependent, homogeneous, echogenic substance without acoustic shadowing in the gallbladder lumen (**Figures 3** and **4**) [17].

4.1.3 Adenomyomatosis

Adenomyomatosis may present as a protuberant lesion or a wall thickening lesion, and in both cases may mimic gallbladder carcinoma. As a protuberant lesion, adenomyomatosis tends to be sessile in nature, with a single or multiple anechoic internal areas (i.e. microcysts) corresponding to Rokitansky-Aschoff sinuses (RAS) (**Figure 5**). The surface is relatively granular and irregular. Some lesions may demonstrate internal echoes with a comet tail artifact due to multipath reflection from RAS or intramural calculi [1, 12]. They tend to appear oval in shape. Although adenomyomatosis are typically benign lesions, cases of co-existing gallbladder carcinoma with adenomyomatosis have been reported [12, 22].

Adenomyomatosis can also appear as focal or diffuse gallbladder wall thickening. Comet tail artifacts and RAS are also present in the wall-thickening lesions. The layers of the gallbladder wall tend to be preserved within the lesion, and the surface is usually smooth in appearance, although in some cases it may feature some degree of irregularity due to mucosal hyperplastic changes [12]. Surface irregularity should raise suspicion for the presence of gallbladder carcinoma within the adenomyomatous lesions [3].

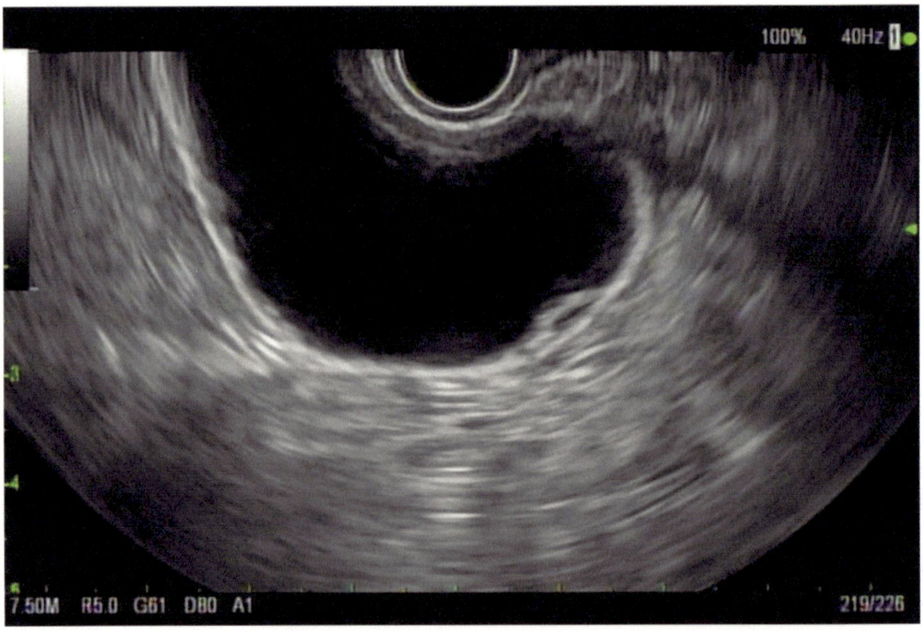

Figure 5.
Protuberant adenomyomatosis with an internal anechoic area representing a Rokitansky-Aschoff sinus.

4.2 Neoplastic protuberant gallbladder lesions

4.2.1 Gallbladder adenoma

Gallbladder adenomas are uncommon and comprise 10% of all gallbladder polyps diagnosed by ultrasound [15]. They are generally homogeneously isoechoic with multiple microcysts within the polyp. They are oval with a relatively smooth surface and may be pedunculated or sub-pedunculated. They typically range from between 5 mm to 20 mm in diameter [3, 12]. On EUS, adenomas are difficult to distinguish from gallbladder carcinoma, but certain distinguishing features such as an intralesional vascular spot on color Doppler investigation or uniform contrast enhancement may aid in differentiating the two [3, 15, 23]. They have malignant potential and are at risk of progressing to gallbladder cancer through the adenoma-carcinoma sequence, although the incidence of this requires further elucidation [3, 24].

4.2.2 Gallbladder carcinoma

Gallbladder carcinoma typically demonstrates invasion of the gallbladder mucosa [25]. They are more commonly sessile than pedunculated, and the internal echo is heterogeneously dense, with increased echogenicity and scattered hypoechoic areas in the core. The outer surface of the carcinoma is typically nodular, and the shape is round [12]. In contrast to cholesterol polyps which tend to become irregular in shape beyond a diameter of 10 mm, carcinomas retain their rounded structure after reaching this size [1]. Prior studies investigating large polyps >10 mm in size, singular polyps >14 mm were 92.3% sensitive for differentiating neoplastic from non-neoplastic polyps, and sessile structure or polyp size >22 mm were 93.5–95.7% sensitive for differentiating carcinomas from adenomas [26]. Kozuka et al. in their examination of surgical gallbladder specimens found that a diameter of 12 mm or greater was associated with cancerous foci, and most invasive carcinomas were greater than 30 mm in diameter [24]. Sessile shape increases the odds of malignancy by a factor of 7.32 [27].

5. Gallbladder wall thickening

Gallbladder wall thickening is defined as a thickness of the gallbladder wall greater than 4 mm. Wall thickening lesions are further classified as local (<50%) or diffuse (>50%) depending on the extent of the involved portion. Furthermore, focal wall thickening may also refer to instances in which there is a focal presence of an inner hypoechoic layer, even if the wall is less than 4 mm thick [11, 12].

Diffuse gallbladder wall thickening is caused by several gallbladder disorders and non-gallbladder disorders, including extra-cholecystic inflammation, liver disease, systemic disease, and pseudo-thickening. However, in comparison, focal gallbladder wall thickening is more specific for intrinsic gallbladder disease and in the context of some diseases such as xanthogranulomatous cholecystitis, is more concerning for gallbladder carcinoma [25, 28].

Thus, although the differential diagnosis of gallbladder wall thickening is broad, in general it can be further classified into diffuse and focal involvement. In some cases, gallbladder wall thickening may be due to malignancy and thus distinguishing these from benign causes is important. EUS features that may assist with delineating this include the contour of the lesion, patterns of the wall thickness, the presence of intramural cystic spaces, and patterns of gallbladder wall enhancement [12].

5.1 Benign gallbladder wall thickening

5.1.1 Adenomyomatosis

See the above section on "Benign Protuberant Gallbladder Lesions."

5.1.2 Cholecystitis

Typical sonographic findings of acute cholecystitis include the presence of gallstones, gallstone impaction in the gallbladder neck or cystic duct, gallbladder distention, gallbladder wall thickening, and pericholecystic fluid [29]. Typical findings on EUS include diffuse gallbladder wall thickening, a smooth inner mucosal layer, and preservation of the gallbladder wall layer structure [12]. However, EUS, at the present, is not the imaging modality of choice for diagnosis of acute cholecystitis, whereas TAUS and CT scan are preferred. The appearance of chronic cholecystitis is similar to that of acute cholecystitis.

Chronic xanthogranulomatous cholecystitis (XGC) is a subtype of chronic cholecystitis characterized by irregular gallbladder wall thickening and fibrosis due to chronic inflammation related to intramural infection. Granulomas form in the gallbladder wall due to the phagocytosis of purulent bile by histiocytes. Known causes of XGC include impaction of stones in the gallbladder neck or leakage of bile into the gallbladder wall due to rupture of RAS or mucosal ulceration. XGC may closely resemble gallbladder carcinoma on EUS and may require biopsy for diagnosis [3, 10, 12]. On EUS, the extent of wall thickening may be focal or diffuse, and the mucosa retains a smooth surface. In some cases, intramural hyperechoic nodules may be present. The wall may demonstrate a mixed hyperechoic and hypoechoic echotexture with irregularity or disruption of the gallbladder wall layers [12].

5.1.3 Other causes of benign gallbladder wall thickening

Other causes of gallbladder wall thickening include pseudothickening, systemic disease, liver disease, or neighboring inflammatory conditions. Focal pseudothickening is associated with the presence of debris and sludge within the gallbladder lumen, whereas diffuse pseudothickening is seen in postprandial states. States of fluid overload or and third-spacing, such as heart failure, renal failure, cirrhosis, hypoalbuminemia, and sepsis are common systemic diseases associated with diffuse gallbladder wall thickening. Inflammation of nearby organs, such as that which occurs during pancreatitis, hepatitis, or peritonitis may also lead to diffuse gallbladder wall thickening [11].

5.2 Neoplastic wall thickening

5.2.1 Gallbladder carcinoma (wall thickening type)

Wall-thickening gallbladder carcinoma is difficult to diagnose based on EUS alone, because it is mimicked by other conditions such as adenomyomatosis and XGC. The examination reveals an irregular or papillated mucosa, and non-uniform wall thickening marked by non-uniform hypoechoic patterns. In addition, the structure of the wall layers is ill-defined and may appear disrupted depending on the depth of invasion. Gallbladder carcinoma is differentiated from adenomyomatosis by the absence of RAS and intramural microcysts. Predictive findings of gallbladder carcinoma may include loss of the multiple layer wall pattern, wall thickness greater than 10 mm, absence of gallstones, and hypoechoic internal echogenicity [12, 30, 31].

6. EUS-guided tissue acquisition

6.1 Introduction

Endoscopic ultrasound-guided fine needle aspiration (FNA) is a useful method for the diagnosis of gallbladder disease. Differentiating malignant from benign gallbladder lesions is important due to the high short term mortality rates of gallbladder carcinoma, and because imaging alone is often insufficient to establish a diagnosis. Obtaining gallbladder tissue to establish a diagnosis is therefore necessary to guide clinical decision-making. Prior techniques such as endoscopic brush biopsy during endoscopic retrograde cholangiopancreatography (ERCP) and endoscopic transpapillary gallbladder drainage (ETP-GBD) were shown to have low sensitivities of 47.4% and 71%, respectively [32, 33]. These methods are technically difficult, and entering the major papilla inherently carries the risks of complications such as post-ERCP pancreatitis, cholangitis, and sepsis [32]. With ETP-GBD in particular, the incidence of these major complications in addition to perforation of the cystic duct is between 0 and 14% [32]. Furthermore, bile duct biopsy using ERCP is unable to provide direct samples of the gallbladder lesion itself, and is primarily indicated when a biliary stricture is present. If a biliary stricture is absent, biliary cytology through ETP-GBD was previously required [10]. Now, EUS-FNA is increasingly being used in the diagnosis and management of pancreaticobiliary lesions, including those of the gallbladder. The diagnostic sensitivities of EUS-FNA exceed that of both ERCP and ETP-GBD [32, 33]. A meta-analysis combining nine studies analyzing the use of EUS-FNA for the diagnosis of gallbladder lesions reported a combined sensitivity of 84%, and other studies have reported specificities of 100% [3, 34–39].

6.2 Current indications

The current use of EUS-FNA of the gallbladder itself from a diagnostic standpoint is mostly limited to gallbladder wall thickening lesions due to paucity of data and concern for complications. In terms of gallbladder cancer, Hijioka et al. propose the use of this procedure for some cases of resectable gallbladder cancer, especially when there is ambiguity about the malignant potential of a lesion or when surgery is considered extremely invasive [3]. EUS-FNA is not recommended for most cases of resectable gallbladder cancer because there is no role for neoadjuvant chemotherapy. Due to the similarity in endoscopic appearance of XGC and gallbladder cancer, EUS-FNA can guide the diagnosis and avoid extensive high-risk surgery for the patient. Nonetheless, they recommend taking EUS-FNA biopsy results with skepticism in some cases of XGC due to the propensity of the disease to co-exist with gallbladder carcinoma in a small percentage of cases [40]. Complete examination of the gallbladder including the neck and cystic duct are recommended, as obstructive gallbladder carcinoma may occur in this area and lead to XGC of the gallbladder body and fundus.

Another technique to differentiate XGC from gallbladder carcinoma involves biopsy of the surrounding lymph nodes [3].

6.3 Complications

Current data on the safety of EUS-FNA of the gallbladder suggest low complication rates. Potential complications of the procedure include cholangitis, bleeding, or bile leak, although several studies report no serious adverse events after the procedure [32, 33, 36]. Although this suggests that EUS-FNA is safe, the possibility of reporting bias necessitates further research to elucidate the potential harms of the procedure [36].

One of the most feared complications of EUS-FNA is the possibility of bile leak as a result of gallbladder perforation, leading to peritoneal dissemination of infection or malignancy [41, 42]. The risk of this may be higher in cases of gallbladder polyps, where biopsy would require traversing the gallbladder lumen, and EUS-FNA should be avoided in such cases [3]. Nonetheless, cases of successful EUS-FNA of gallbladder intraluminal lesions have been reported [37, 38, 43]. Wall thickening lesions usually carry a lower risk of gallbladder perforation because the needle tract may travel tangentially with respect to the gallbladder, and as such are more amenable to EUS-FNA. The risk of needle tract seeding leading to intragastric metastases may be increased in EUS-FNA, although the occurrence of this is rare [44, 45]. Alternative sites than the gallbladder itself should be surveyed for metastatic disease, such as the liver or neighboring lymph nodes, as these are usually safer to biopsy. According to some authors, the portion of the gallbladder wall that makes contact with the liver parenchyma is a technically preferred location for biopsy [10].

6.4 EUS-FNB

EUS-FNA with rapid onsite evaluation of cytopathology (ROSE) is the current preferred approach to tissue sampling of pancreaticobiliary lesions due to a high diagnostic yield of greater than 90% [46]. However, this method is not without limitations; it requires considerable expertise, personnel, and resources, and is unavailable outside of most tertiary care centers. Another disadvantage is that it relies on adequate cellularity of the sample, where in some cases if a lesion is significantly fibrotic or necrotic the diagnostic yield is poor [47].

Novel fine needle biopsy (FNB) devices were developed for use with EUS and have produced optimistic results. Specifically, the development of the fork-tip needle (SharkCore, Medtronic, USA) in 2016 and the Franseen tip needle (Acquire, Boston Scientific, USA) in 2017 have allowed endosonographers to perform endoscopic biopsies with excellent diagnostic yield. A striking benefit of FNB is that it allows for the acquisition of larger tissue samples that can be analyzed histopathologically, potentially obviating the need for EUS-FNA with ROSE. Emerging studies on FNB in pancreaticobiliary lesions other than that of the gallbladder have shown promising results. Adequate tissue acquisition rates with the Franseen tip needle were reported to be greater than 90% in one multicenter study [48]. A recent meta-analysis demonstrated that the addition of ROSE did not improve the diagnostic accuracy of FNB [49]. Randomized controlled trials have demonstrated diagnostic accuracies of greater than 90% with both FNB needle types, and a subsequent multicenter randomized controlled trial showed that the diagnostic accuracy of FNB was non-inferior to EUS-FNA with ROSE [47, 50, 51]. Furthermore, FNB was associated with fewer needle passes, shorter procedure times, and comparable associated costs when compared to EUS-FNA with ROSE [47]. Yet, the use of FNB for gallbladder lesions remains uncommon, with limited data available reporting both high diagnostic accuracy and safety in the context of gallbladder lesions [43, 52]. The development of large multicenter trials focusing on the use of FNB in gallbladder lesions is necessary to guide future indications for this technique.

Another perk to FNB is that in the retrieval of larger tissue volumes, this permits histopathological analysis by immunohistochemistry, and in turn, empowers diagnostic capabilities by introducing next-generation genetic sequencing. Several potential targetable genes have already been identified in gallbladder carcinoma and cholangiocarcinoma, and trials specifically targeting HER2-positive cholangiocarcinoma are currently underway [53–55]. The treatment landscape of gallbladder and biliary tract cancer is fairly young, but there is optimism that FNB will become increasingly useful in advancing our ability to identify targeted therapies for gallbladder cancers.

7. Conclusion

Endoscopic ultrasound is an essential tool in the evaluation of biliary disease. The gallbladder examination from an endoscopic point of view provides clinicians with a unique advantage in identifying pathology that may be difficult to visualize by other imaging modalities such as cross-sectional imaging and TAUS. However, this technique does have limitations, namely in its ability to distinguish gallbladder polypoid lesions and to ascertain malignant lesions from those that are benign. Tissue diagnosis is often required, which is in some cases achievable by EUS as well. EUS-guided tissue acquisition has propelled our diagnostic capabilities of gallbladder and other pancreaticobiliary lesions and paved bright avenues toward the possibility of targeted treatments in the future.

Conflict of interest

The authors declare no conflict of interest.

Author details

Landon Kozai[1] and Larissa Fujii-Lau[2]*

1 University of Hawai'i, Honolulu, Hawaii, USA

2 The Queen's Medical Center, Honolulu, Hawaii, USA

*Address all correspondence to: llau@queens.org

References

[1] Azuma T, Yoshikawa T, Araida T, Takasaki K. Differential diagnosis of polypoid lesions of the gallbladder by endoscopic ultrasonography. American Journal of Surgery. 2001;**181**(1):65-70

[2] Sugiyama M, Atomi Y, Yamato T. Endoscopic ultrasonography for differential diagnosis of polypoid gall bladder lesions: Analysis in surgical and follow up series. Gut. 2000;**46**(2):250

[3] Hijioka S, Nagashio Y, Ohba A, Maruki Y, Okusaka T. The role of EUS and EUS-FNA in differentiating benign and malignant gallbladder lesions. Diagnostics. 2021;**11**(9):1586

[4] Ellis H. Anatomy of the gallbladder and bile ducts. Surgery (Oxford). 2011;**29**(12):593-596

[5] Sharma M, Somani P, Sunkara T. Imaging of gall bladder by endoscopic ultrasound. World Journal of Gastrointestinal Endoscopy. 2018;**10**(1):10-15

[6] Okada KI, Kijima H, Imaizumi T, Hirabayashi K, Matsuyama M, Yazawa N, et al. Wall-invasion pattern correlates with survival of patients with gallbladder adenocarcinoma. Anticancer Research. 2009;**29**(2):685-691

[7] Wang JY, Mu PY, Xu YK, Bai YY, Shen DH. Application of imaging techniques in pancreaticobiliary maljunction. World Journal of Clinical Cases. 2022;**10**(22):7642-7652

[8] Fujita N, Noda Y, Kobayashi G, Kimura K, Yago A, Mochizuki F. Analysis of the layer structure of the Gallbladder Wall delineated by endoscopic ultrasound using the pinning method. Digestive Endoscopy. 1995;7(4):353-356

[9] Watanabe Y, Goto H, Naitoh Y, Hirooka Y, Itoh A, Taki T, et al. Usefulness of intraductal ultrasonography in gallbladder disease. Journal of Ultrasound in Medicine. 1998;**17**(1):33-39

[10] Tanaka K, Katanuma A, Hayashi T, Kin T, Takahashi K. Role of -endoscopic ultrasound for gallbladder disease. Journal of Medical Ultrasonics. 2021;**48**(2):187-198

[11] Okaniwa S. How can we manage gallbladder lesions by transabdominal ultrasound? Diagnostics. 2021;**11**(5):784

[12] Hashimoto S, Nakaoka K, Kawabe N, Kuzuya T, Funasaka K, Nagasaka M, et al. The role of endoscopic ultrasound in the diagnosis of gallbladder lesions. Diagnostics. 2021;**11**(10):1789

[13] Choi JH, Seo DW, Choi JH, Park DH, Lee SS, Lee SK, et al. Utility of contrast-enhanced harmonic EUS in the diagnosis of malignant gallbladder polyps (with videos). Gastrointestinal Endoscopy. 2013;**78**(3):484-493

[14] Andrén-Sandberg Å. Diagnosis and management of gallbladder polyps. North American Journal of Medical Sciences. 2012;**4**(5):203-211

[15] Cocco G, Basilico R, Pizzi AD, Cocco N, Boccatonda A, D'Ardes D, et al. Gallbladder polyps ultrasound: What the sonographer needs to know. Journal of Ultrasound. 2021;**24**(2):131-142

[16] Thorbøll J, Vilmann P, Jacobsen B, Hassan H. Endoscopic ultrasonography in detection of cholelithiasis in patients with biliary pain and negative transabdominal ultrasonography.

World Journal of Gastroenterology. 2004;**39**(3):267-269

[17] Somani P, Sunkara T, Sharma M. Role of endoscopic ultrasound in idiopathic pancreatitis. World Journal of Gastroenterology. 2017;**23**(38):6952-6961

[18] Pereira R, Eslick G, Cox M. Endoscopic ultrasound for routine assessment in idiopathic acute pancreatitis. Journal of Gastrointestinal Surgery. 2019;**23**(8):1694-1700

[19] Valverde-López F, Ortega-Suazo EJ, Wilcox CM, Cano MCF, Martínez-Cara JG, Redondo-Cerezo E. Endoscopic ultrasound as a diagnostic and predictive tool in idiopathic acute pancreatitis. Annals of Gastroenterology. 2020;**33**(3):305-312

[20] Kondo S, Isayama H, Akahane M, Toda N, Sasahira N, Nakai Y, et al. Detection of common bile duct stones: Comparison between endoscopic ultrasonography, magnetic resonance cholangiography, and helical-computed-tomographic cholangiography. European Journal of Radiology. 2005;**54**(2):271-275

[21] Vila J, Mendioroz F, Yeaton P, Fernández-Urién I, Sanchotena J, Goñi S, et al. EUS is superior to secretin-enhanced cholangio-MRI to establish the etiology of idiopathic acute pancreatitis. Endoscopy International Open. 2020;**08**(10):E1441-E1447

[22] Nabatame N, Shirai Y, Nishimura A, Yokoyama N, Wakai T, Hatakeyama K. High risk of gallbladder carcinoma in elderly patients with segmental adenomyomatosis of the gallbladder. Journal of Experimental & Clinical Cancer Research. 2004;**23**(4):593-598

[23] Park CH, Chung MJ, Oh TG, Park JY, Bang S, Park SW, et al. Differential diagnosis between gallbladder adenomas and cholesterol polyps on contrast-enhanced harmonic endoscopic ultrasonography. Surgical Endoscopy. 2013;**27**(4):1414-1421

[24] Kozuka S, Tsubone M, Yasui A, Hachisuka K. Relation of adenoma to carcinoma in the gallbladder. Cancer. 1982;**50**(10):2226-2234

[25] Okaniwa S. Everything you need to know about ultrasound for diagnosis of gallbladder diseases. Journal of Medical Ultrasonics. 2021;**48**(2):145-147

[26] Choi TW, Kim JH, Park SJ, Ahn SJ, Joo I, Han JK. Risk stratification of gallbladder polyps larger than 10 mm using high-resolution ultrasonography and texture analysis. European Radiology. 2018;**28**(1):196-205

[27] Bhatt NR, Gillis A, Smoothey CO, Awan FN, Ridgway PF. Evidence based management of polyps of the gall bladder: A systematic review of the risk factors of malignancy. Surg. 2016;**14**(5):278-286

[28] Cui Y, Zhang H, Zhao E, Cui N, Li Z. Differential diagnosis and treatment options for Xanthogranulomatous cholecystitis. Medical Principles and Practice. 2012;**22**(1):18-23

[29] Oppenheimer DC, Rubens DJ. Sonography of acute cholecystitis and its mimics. Radiologic Clinics of North America. 2019;**57**(3):535-548

[30] Kim HJ, Park JH, Park DI, Cho YK, Sohn CI, Jeon WK, et al. Clinical usefulness of endoscopic ultrasonography in the differential diagnosis of Gallbladder Wall thickening. Digestive Diseases and Sciences. 2012;**57**(2):508-515

[31] Mizuguchi M, Kudo S, Fukahori T, Matsuo Y, Miyazaki K, Tokunaga O,

et al. Endoscopic ultrasonography for demonstrating loss of multiple-layer pattern of the thickened gallbladder wall in the preoperative diagnosis of gallbladder cancer. European Radiology. 1997;**7**(8):1323-1327

[32] Ogura T, Kurisu Y, Masuda D, Imoto A, Onda S, Kamiyama R, et al. Can endoscopic ultrasound-guided fine needle aspiration offer clinical benefit for thick-walled gallbladders? Digestive Diseases and Sciences. 2014;**59**(8):1917-1924

[33] Hijioka S, Hara K, Mizuno N, Imaoka H, Ogura T, Haba S, et al. Diagnostic yield of endoscopic retrograde cholangiography and of EUS-guided fine needle aspiration sampling in gallbladder carcinomas. Journal of Hepato-Biliary-Pancreatic Sciences. 2012;**19**(6):650-655

[34] Wu LM, Jiang XX, Gu HY, Xu X, Zhang W, Lin LH, et al. Endoscopic ultrasound-guided fine-needle aspiration biopsy in the evaluation of bile duct strictures and gallbladder masses. European Journal of Gastroenterology & Hepatology. 2011;**23**(2):113-120

[35] Hijioka S, Mekky MA, Bhatia V, Sawaki A, Mizuno N, Hara K, et al. Can EUS-guided FNA distinguish between gallbladder cancer and xanthogranulomatous cholecystitis? Gastrointestinal Endoscopy. 2010;**72**(3):622-627

[36] Singla V, Agarwal R, Anikhindi S, Puri P, Kumar M, Ranjan P, et al. Role of EUS-FNA for gallbladder mass lesions with biliary obstruction: A large single-center experience. Endoscopy International Open. 2019;**07**(11):E1403-E1409

[37] Jacobson BC, Pitman MB, Brugge WR. EUS-guided FNA for the diagnosis of gallbladder masses. Gastrointestinal Endoscopy. 2003;**57**(2):251-254

[38] Varadarajulu S, Eloubeidi M. Endoscopic ultrasound-guided fine-needle aspiration in the evaluation of gallbladder masses. Endoscopy. 2005;**37**(8):751-754

[39] Meara RS, Jhala D, Eloubeidi MA, Eltoum I, Chhieng DC, Crowe DR, et al. Endoscopic ultrasound-guided FNA biopsy of bile duct and gallbladder: Analysis of 53 cases. Cytopathology. 2006;**17**(1):42-49

[40] Lee HS, Joo KR, Kim DH, Park NH, Jeong YK, Suh JH, et al. A case of simultaneous Xanthogranulomatous cholecystitis and carcinoma of the gallbladder. The Korean Journal of Internal Medicine. 2003;**18**(1):53-56

[41] Kojima H, Kitago M, Iwasaki E, Masugi Y, Matsusaka Y, Yagi H, et al. Peritoneal dissemination of pancreatic cancer caused by endoscopic ultrasound-guided fine needle aspiration: A case report and literature review. World Journal of Gastroenterology. 2021;**27**(3):294-304

[42] Hirooka Y, Goto H, Itoh A, Hashimoto S, Niwa K, IshiKAwa H, et al. Case of intraductal papillary mucinous tumor in which Endosonography-guided fine-needle aspiration biopsy caused dissemination. European Journal of Gastroenterology & Hepatology. 2003;**18**(11):1323-1324

[43] Kang SH, Joo JS, Kim SH, Kim KH, Lee ES. EUS-guided fine-needle biopsy of gallbladder polypoid lesions. Videogie. 2020;**5**(4):151-153

[44] Ngamruengphong S, Xu C, Woodward T, Raimondo M, Stauffer J, Asbun H, et al. Risk of gastric

or peritoneal recurrence, and long-term outcomes, following pancreatic cancer resection with preoperative endosonographically guided fine needle aspiration. Endoscopy. 2013;**45**(08):619-626

[45] Dumonceau JM, Deprez P, Jenssen C, Iglesias-Garcia J, Larghi A, Vanbiervliet G, et al. Indications, results, and clinical impact of endoscopic ultrasound (EUS)-guided sampling in gastroenterology: European Society of Gastrointestinal Endoscopy (ESGE) clinical guideline – Updated January 2017. Endoscopy. 2017;**49**(07):695-714

[46] Hammoud GM, Almashhrawi A, Ibdah JA. Usefulness of endoscopic ultrasound-guided fine needle aspiration in the diagnosis of hepatic, gallbladder and biliary tract lesions. World Journal of Gastrointestinal Oncology. 2014;**6**(11):420

[47] Chen YI, Chatterjee A, Berger R, Kanber Y, Wyse J, Lam E, et al. Endoscopic ultrasound (EUS)-guided fine needle biopsy alone vs. EUS-guided fine needle aspiration with rapid onsite evaluation in pancreatic lesions: A multicenter randomized trial. Endoscopy. 2022;**54**(01):4-12

[48] Adler DG, Muthusamy VR, Ehrlich DS, Parasher G, Thosani NC, Chen A, et al. A multicenter evaluation of a new EUS core biopsy needle: Experience in 200 patients. Endoscopic Ultrasound. 2019;**8**(2):99-104

[49] Facciorusso A, Gkolfakis P, Tziatzios G, Ramai D, Papanikolaou IS, Triantafyllou K, et al. Comparison between EUS-guided fine-needle biopsy with or without rapid on-site evaluation for tissue sampling of solid pancreatic lesions: A systematic review and meta-analysis. Endoscopic Ultrasound. 2022;**11**(6):458-465

[50] Bang JY, Hebert-Magee S, Navaneethan U, Hasan MK, Hawes R, VaradarajuluS.Randomizedtrialcomparing the Franseen and fork-tip needles for EUS-guided fine-needle biopsy sampling of solid pancreatic mass lesions. Gastrointestinal Endoscopy. 2018;**87**(6):1432-1438

[51] Ashat M, Klair JS, Rooney SL, Vishal SJ, Jensen C, Sahar N, et al. Randomized controlled trial comparing the Franseen needle with the fork-tip needle for EUS-guided fine-needle biopsy. Gastrointestinal Endoscopy. 2021;**93**(1):140-150.e2

[52] Tong T, Tian L, Deng MZ, Chen XJ, Fu T, Ma KJ, et al. The efficacy and safety of endoscopic ultrasound-guided fine-needle biopsy in gallbladder masses. Hepatobiliary & Pancreatic Diseases International. 2022

[53] Shibata T, Arai Y, Totoki Y. Molecular genomic landscapes of hepatobiliary cancer. Cancer Science. 2018;**109**(5):1282-1291

[54] Javle M, Borad MJ, Azad NS, Kurzrock R, Abou-Alfa GK, George B, et al. Pertuzumab and trastuzumab for HER2-positive, metastatic biliary tract cancer (MyPathway): A multicentre, open-label, phase 2a, multiple basket study. The Lancet Oncology. 2021;**22**(9):1290-1300

[55] Hirata K, Kuwatani M, Suda G, Ishikawa M, Sugiura R, Kato S, et al. A novel approach for the genetic analysis of biliary tract cancer specimens obtained through endoscopic ultrasound-guided fine needle aspiration using targeted amplicon sequencing. Clinical and Translational Gastroenterology. 2019;**10**(3):e00022

Chapter 4

Diet and Gallstone

Reginald del Pozo

Abstract

Cholesterol gallstone disease is a major health problem in western countries and depends on genetic and enviromental factors. Diet may influence the formation of gallstone either by altering the biliary lipid composition or by modifying gallbladder motility. Numerous investigations have examined the association of diet and cholesterol gallstone in prospective, cross-sectional, and case-control studies and in experimental animal models. However, these findings are controversial, probably because human studies are mainly epidemiological with differences in study designs, dietary exposure assessment, and methods used. In general, a high intake of saturated fats and refined sugars has been shown to increase the risk of forming cholesterol gallstones, while a high intake of monounsaturated fats and fiber may decrease this process. The pathogenic mechanisms behind these alterations are reviewed, and the need for a nutritional intervention based on a diet low in lipids and rich in fibers is highlighted. A better understanding of the role of diet in gallstone formation may provide tools for those patients who have been diagnosed with symptomatic gallstones and may also contribute to the prophylactic and therapeutic strategies for cholelithiasis.

Keywords: dietary impact, gallbladder disease, gallstones, nutrition, risk factors

1. Introduction

Cholesterol gallstone disease is a very common pathology in western populations, with a high global prevalence of approximately 10–20%. The etiology of this pathology is considered multifactorial depending on the interaction of numerous complex factors: obesity, dyslipidemia, insulin resistance, high consumption of refined carbohydrates and cholesterol, age, female sex hormones, ethnicity, and sedentary lifestyles [1–3]. Pathological conditions result from a rapid and large mobilization of body cholesterol to the liver and then to the bile. This situation may cause biliary cholesterol supersaturation, increased cholesterol crystallization, and gallbaldder stasis [4]. The relationship between the secretion of bile acids and either phospholipids or free cholesterol represents important ratios of the secreted molecules, usually causing disturbances that result in a lithogenic bile [5]. The main risk factors in the pathogenesis of gallstones are biliary cholesterol hypersaturation, cholesterol crystallization, cholesterol crystal agglomeration and growth, and gallbladder dysmotility [6, 7]. The relationships between bile acid secretion and free cholesterol are highly species-dependent and, within certain species, are easily affected by diet. However, not all species present biliary characteristics required for cholesterol crystallization and stone formation, such as bile stasis, sludge formation, and nucleating factors, after cholesterol supersaturation is reached [8]. The use of animal models is limited because relatively few species always develop gallstones, and unlike humans, they do not spontaneously generate supersaturated bile in the gallbladder [9]. Therefore, there are certain contradictions in clinical and research studies, whose conclusions should be carefully analyzed. Another difficulty inherent in these studies is the impossibility of knowing the onset time of the disease caused by a specific dietary factor, in addition to not knowing the exact dimension of energy intake and the estimation of the dietary constituents effectively ingested [10].

Many epidemiological studies have associated the formation of cholesterol gallstones with other pathologies such as obesity, hyperlipidemia, and type 2 diabetes mellitus [11–13]. The presence of multiple risk factors in common with other disease makes it possible to associate gallstone disease with other cardiovascular diseases such as atherosclerosis carotid disease and metabolic dysfunction [14]. Although cholesterol gallstones genesis is multifactorial, basic physiological correlates associated with dietary modulation of biliary lipid metabolism are discussed in relation to gallstone disease. Several investigations have reported on the role of specific dietary constituents as a potential risk factor for cholelithiasis. Diet may influence the formation of gallstones either by modifying gallbladder motility or by altering the biliary lipid composition. The importance of diet in the pathogenesis of gallstones has been much debated. Most of these epidemiological investigations correspond to prospective, cross-sectional, or case-control studies. Some studies show specific nutrients that promote and others that, on the contrary, protect the process of gallstone formation [15]. Among the many dietary factors suggested in the literature, we will focus mainly on total energy intake, intake of carbohydrates, proteins, total fats, saturated fats, mono- and polyunsaturated fats, cholesterol, total fiber, and alcohol. Evidence on the relation between diet and gallstone formation, however, is somewhat conflicting.

The aim of this chapter is to present experimental and epidemiological evidence of dietetic factors that may favor the process of cholesterol gallstone formation.

2. Specific role of various dietary components

A number of dietary factors have been involved in the pathogenesis of cholesterol gallstone formation (**Figure 1**). It has been reported that Western-type diets, hypercaloric, high in fat and refined sugars, and limited intake of fiber, are factors that increase the possibility of gallstone formation. It is relevant to review nutritional factors that impact the relationship between the relative flow of cholesterol through bile lipids, which constitutes a crucial event in the process of the formation of cholesterol gallstones. Consequently, diet appears to alter most of the components secreted into the bile.

2.1 Obesity and caloric intake

An excess in energy intake has been related to an increased risk of developing cholelithiasis. Obesity represents the greatest risk factor for cholelthiasis, since it exhibits an increase in the bile secretion of cholesterol from the liver, which generates cholesterol supersaturated bile; crystallization of cholesterol monohydrates; and agglomeration and growth until macroscopic gallstones formation [16, 17]. This excess cholesterol is secreted by hepatocytes as a direct result of increased body

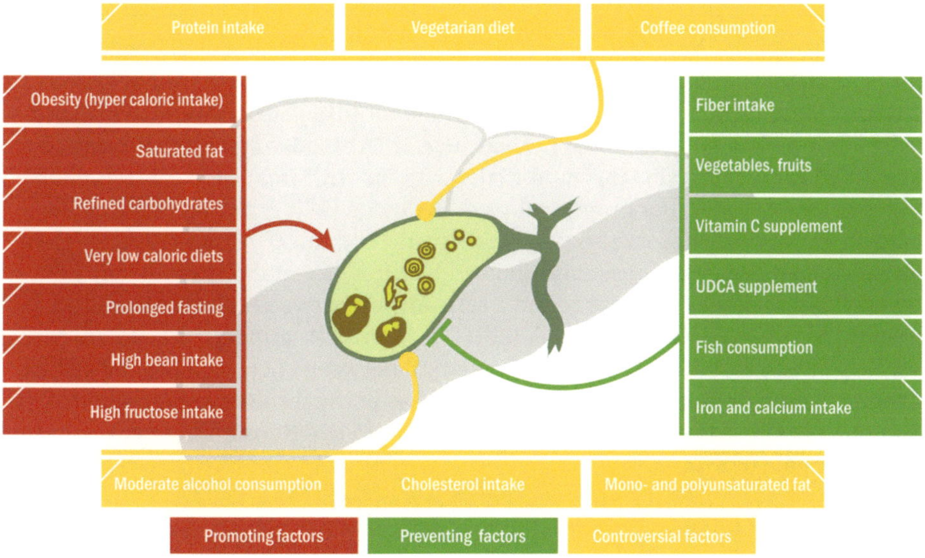

Figure 1.
Effects of major dietary factors (promoting-, preventing- and controversial factors) on gallstone formation.

weight. It has been estimated that each extra kilogram of body fat yields the production of approximately 20 mg of additional cholesterol [12, 18]. A relevant factor in the process of the formation of cholesterol gallstones is the relative mass of free cholesterol in the bile, which is associated with the consumption of an overload of calories in the diet. Probably the link between obesity and gallstones reflects an excessive production of cholesterol or an increase in its efflux, which are greatly increased both in nonobese and obese patients with this disease [19]. It has recently been reported that high concentrations of C-reactive protein (CRP) could be an independent risk factor that could trigger the process of gallstone formation [20]. It is unknown how an increase in CRP increases the risk of gallstones, but it is suggested that the secretion of the proinflammatory cytokine interleukin-6 is stimulated by adipose tissue, promoting systemic inflammation in obesity [21, 22]. Many case-control studies have examined the relationship between energy intake and the prevalence of gallstone disease, but the findings are controversial. A French study showed a high risk of gallstone disease in men consuming a high-calorie diet, greater than 2500 Kcal per day, but not in women [23]. Similarly, a Spanish study showed a higher consumption of total calories and fat in patients with gallstones compared to healthy controls [24]. In addition, a prospective study (88,837 controls and 612 symptomatic gallstones patients) reported a positive correlation between energy intake and cholelithiasis [18]. Also, another Mendelian randomization study in 77,679 individuals revealed that an increased BMI caused a link with a risk of symptomatic stones [25]. The distribution of body fat also affects the risk of gallstone, with prospective cohort studies showing an association between gallstone formation and central adiposity compared to lower extremity adiposity [26]. An increase in BMI with high waist circumference and central adiposity can influence the key steps involved in the cholesterol gallstone pathogenesis, particularly an increase in biliary cholesterol concentrations [27, 28]. In addition, obese people frequently show a greater fasting gallbladder volume and a decrease in postprandial gallbladder emptying, which are factors that promote gallstones formation [29, 30].

Generally, a weight loss reduces the risk of gallstones, but an excessive weight loss (greater than 25% of body weight) or undergoing bariatric surgery increases the risk of triggering gallstones [31–33]. The administration of ursodeoxycholic acid during loss of weight could prevent the development of lithogenic changes in bile and the formation of gallstones [34–37]. Treatment with ursodeoxycholic acid should be reserved for the occasional symptomatic patients with small stones presumably formed from cholesterol or proven gallbladder sludge [38]. A retrospective cross-sectional Asian study observed participants younger than 50 years to have a higher risk gallstone if they were obese and showed features of metabolic syndrome [39]. However, other studies have not found a relationship between caloric intake and cholelithiasis [40, 41]. In contrast, an Italian large cross-sectional, ultrasound-based study reported a significant negative association between energy intake and risk of gallstone disease in men [42]. These discrepancies in the results can be explained by differences in the study design and the methods used to determine energy intake and to diagnose gallstone disease.

2.2 Dietary fatty acids

The role of total dietary fat as an etiologic factor for cholelithiasis has been extensively studied but remains unresolved. The overall impact of dietary total fat on bile lipids in humans is controversial, where the degree of fat saturation itself has been examined for its influence on lithogenesis with ambiguous results. It has been suggested that the type of dietary fat habitually consumed can influence bile composition in humans. In gallbladder, this influence was noted in the presence of more concentrated bile in the olive oil group. However, this was not translated into a modification of cholesterol saturation, which is likely due to the fact that cholesterol gallstones were present by the time the dietary intervention started [43]. Some epidemiological studies did not find a significant positive correlation between total fat intake and the risk of gallstone disease [18, 41, 44], but other studies showed that patients with gallstones consume more total fat, preferably saturated fatty acids. A cross-sectional Danish study reported a positive, but nonsignificant, correlation between total fat consumption, mainly saturated fatty acids, and gallstone disease detected by ultrasound [40]. Another study also reported a positive correlation between symptomatic cholelithiasis and saturated fat intake [23]. A high intake of saturated fat has been also documented in patients from Southern Italy with incident gallstones detected by ultrasound, as compared to controls [45]. Another article showed that a high-fat diet in Balb/c mice, composed mainly of saturated fatty acids, significantly increased biliary cholesterol concentration, without modifying biliary phospholipids concentration [46]. This biliary cholesterol saturation caused an increase in cholesterol concentration in vesicular transporters. Furthermore, an increase in the cholesterol/phospholipid ratio of vesicular transporters was observed in the bile of animals treated with a high-fat diet. These cholesterol-rich vesicular transporters can aggregate and fuse, favoring the cholesterol crystals formation.

It has also been found that a diet rich in trans fatty acids could promote the formation of cholesterol gallstones [47]. Otherwise, consumption of cis-unsaturated fats was reported to have a protective effect in a prospective cohort study [48]. The effect of monounsaturated fatty acids (MUFA) is more contradictory. A study in hamsters reported that a diet rich in MUFAs may decrease the risk of gallstone formation, relative to saturated fats [49]. Other studies showed that patients with gallstone disease consumed more total lipids, mainly saturated fatty acids [24, 50]. But other case-control study found a protective effect of MUFAs on gallstone formation [45]. No significant differences in biliary lithogenicity were reported in normal persons consuming two lipid-lowering diets: one rich in polyunsaturated fatty acids (PUFAs) and the other rich in oleic acid [51].

It was found that a medical combination of ω-3 PUFAs (EPA and DHA) originating from fish oil had a preventive effect against cholesterol gallstone formation in C57BL/6 J mice [52]. Dietary fish oil supplementation decreases hypertriglyceridemia and reduces cholesterol crystal nucleation along with decreased gallstone formation in prairie dogs [53, 54]. In another study, it was found that the administration of a fish oil diet rich in n-3 PUFA to patients with gallstones decreased biliary cholesterol saturation, although without altering cholesterol crystallization time [55]. Dietary n-3 PUFA supplementation was also shown to have a beneficial effect on bile lithogenicity and bile composition in obese women during weight los [56]. These results suggest that n-3 PUFAs supplementation of obese woman on weight reduction treatment maintains the cholesterol saturation index and cholesterol nucleation time, which might prevent the formation of cholesterol gallstones. Various mechanisms may explain the inhibitory effect of fish oil on gallstone formation: reduction in biliary cholesterol saturation, decrease in cholesterol crystallization due to changes in bile phospholipid composition, and reduction in bile protein concentration [55, 57].

Other studies recommended increased nut consumption to decrease the risk of gallstone occurrence [58, 59]. A large prospective cohort study based on the Nurses' Health Study reported that frequent nut consumption was associated with a lower risk of cholecystectomy in women [60]. Men who consumed nuts five times or more per week appeared to have an approximately 30% lower risk of gallstone disease [59]. Nuts are mostly unsaturated fats [60, 61], a rich source of dietary fiber [60], and have beneficial effects on blood cholesterol and lipoprotein profiles [58].

2.3 Dietary sterols

It is believed that a high cholesterol intake is a predisposing factor to the formation of gallstones. However, epidemiological studies have shown inconclusive results. The experimental consumption of cholesterol by men tends to increase the relative biliary cholesterol concentration and decrease the moles percent of bile acids in both normal subjects [62, 63] and persons with gallstones [62]. Feeding a cholesterol-cholic acid rich diet induces gallstone formation in mice [64]. Feeding excessive cholesterol (>0.85 mg/kcal or 2 g/day human equivalent) is essencially the only way to regularly induce gallstones in most animal model [65]. Under these conditions, bile is typically enriched with cholesterol and reduced in bile acids. A possible mechanism would be that inhibition of hepatic cholesterol synthesis impairs bile acid production in a manner similar to the coordinated inhibition of both cholesterol and bile acid synthesis by lovastatin in humans, while apoE-rich lipoproteins distribute excess absorbed cholesterol directly into the bile [66]. In contrast, other study found no significant increase in biliary cholesterol saturation after 1 month of cholesterol feeding to chickens, rabbits, and rats [67]. Exposure to low dietary cholesterol intake can lead to increased cholesterol synthesis and cholesterol flux into the bile, causing supersaturated bile and thereby increasing the likelihood of forming cholesterol gallstones [10]. These contradictory results may relate to the inclusion of populations from different ethnic groups, with different genetic predisposition and diets, rather than to the effects of cholesterol itself [68].

Plant sterols in diet have been associated with cholesterol gallstone pathogenesis. It was reported that β-sitosterol (a plant sterol present in corn oil, soy, and bran) prevents gallstone formation in mice fed with a lithogenic diet, by decreasing intestinal cholesterol absorption [69]. More recently, a study has demonstrated that plant sterols could inhibit intestinal cholesterol absorption and thus prevent cholesterol gallstone formation [70]. Plant steroids, like diosgenin and other sapogenins, induce massive secretion of cholesterol into rat bile [71]. Legumes that contain significant amounts of sapogenins increase biliary cholesterol saturation and secretion in men and simultaneously decrease serum LDL cholesterol concentration [72, 73]. It is known that the Pima Indians consume large amounts of beans and have one of the highest prevalences of gallstones in the world, a situation that is common with the Chilean Mapuche Indians [10].

2.4 Dietary carbohydrates

Several studies have evaluated the effect of carbohydrates and have revealed that consumption of refined sugars is directly associated with gallbladder disease [40, 41, 45, 74–76]. Reducing energy-dense foods, particularly those high in sugar, has shown beneficial effects on both weight and gallstone risk [77]. A prospective study found a significant association between increasing total dietary glycemic load and the subsequent risk of cholecystectomy in women, indicating that both the quality and quantity of carbohydrate intake is important in predicting risk of cholecystectomy [78]. The effect of a high carbohydrate on gallstone risk have been confirmed by a large ultrasonographic study in pregnant women [79]. Women were assessed for dietary habits, and the risk of incident biliary sludge/gallstones during pregnancy was significantly higher among women in the highest quartile of total carbohydrate intake compared with those in the lower quartiles. Another research group concludes that dietary carbohydrates may play a role in cholesterol gallstone formation by altering biliary motility and by enhancing crystal formation. They suggest that a high carbohydrate diet decreases gallbladder volume, shortens cholesterol crystal observation time, and increases crystal mass [80].

Fructose consumption has dramatically increased in past few decades, is mainly consumed through added sugars (sucrose and high fructose corn syrup), and represents up to 10% of total energy in the US and in several European countries [81, 82]. Many studies have assessed the effects of diets providing large amounts of fructose on various species. The general conclusions from these studies are that a high fructose intake almost invariably leads to increased total energy intake, body weight gain, increased plasma triglyceride concentrations, hepatic and extrahepatic insulin resistance, and diabetes mellitus [83–85]. High intake of fructose (but not sucrose, lactose or galactose) was associated with an increased risk of incident biliary sludge/gallstones, and this association was independent from total carbohydrate intake [79]. The lithogenic effect of fructose appears to depend from several concurrent mechanisms, as induction of insulin resistance, visceral adiposity, metabolic syndrome [86–91], fatty liver secondary to triglycerides accumulation [92], and gallbladder stasis [80]. The deleterious effects of excess fructose intake can produce gastrointestinal symptoms due to intolerance and intestinal fermentation by resident intestinal microbiota [93] and can affect several liver metabolic pathways (gluconeogenesis, glycerol synthesis, and *de novo* lipogenesis) [27]. However, other investigations concluded that there is no clear or convincing evidence that any dietary or added sugar has a unique or detrimental impact on the development of obesity or diabetes compared to any other source of calories [94, 95]. It has been recently reported that fructose apparently does not alter the gallstone formation process in Balb/c mice. Changes in plasma, liver, and bile lipids were only observed at very high fructose concentrations diets [96]. The discrepancies in the results with dietary fructose can be explained because an inadequate consideration is often given to the dose at which these effects occur [97] and also because the metabolic effects of fructose differ between individuals based on their genetic background, suggesting heterogeneity in metabolic responses to dietary fructose in humans [98].

2.5 Dietary protein

Dietary protein as a risk modulator for gallbladder disease has been explored with mixed results. Many animal studies have shown a reduction in gallstones, reduced biliary cholesterol and lithogenic index level [99–103], and lower crystallization rates [104] with higher vegetable protein intake compared to animal protein-rich diets. Human feeding studies examining associations between type (vegetable vs. animal) and quantity of protein and gallbladder disease are limited. Epidemiological studies have observed that people consuming vegetarian diets have a lower incidence of gallbladder disease [105–107], but specific aspects of the vegetarian diet were not fully elucidated. The studies that probe for associated risks between protein intake and gallbladder disease are conflicting. In the prospective Nurses' Health Study, women with increased vegetable protein consumption had reduced risk of developing symptomatic gallstones [108] and lower risk for cholecystectomy [109], but two case-control studies [45, 106] and one other prospective cohort study [42] found no association between gallbladder disease and protein intake. A more recent study has measured the associations between gallbladder disease and protein intake patterns, separated by quantity and type (vegetable vs. animal), among postmenopausal women [110]. They concluded that vegetable protein intake is inversely associated with gallbladder disease risk in postmenopausal women. In addition to weight management, healthcare providers could emphasize vegetable protein as an additional dietary modality to promote lower risk for gallbladder disease. In general, the results suggest that the intake of origin and composition of dietary proteins might be more important than total protein intake in gallstone disease risk.

2.6 Dietary fiber

Dietary fiber includes a wide array of complex substances commonly divided into soluble and insoluble components. Some observational studies have illustrated an inverse relationship between dietary fiber intake and the prevalence of gallstones [111, 112]. Another study investigating the effect of diet as a risk factor for cholesterol gallstone disease implicated that lower dietary fiber and higher refined sugar intake were associated with propensity of gallstone formation [10]. Another study shows a protective effect of dietary soluble fiber against cholesterol gallstone formation [113]. In addition, a large number of epidemiological studies have reported an inverse association between insoluble dietary fiber and gallstone disease [40, 41]. In general, by decreasing the intestinal transit time, dietary fibers may reduce the persistence of bacteria located in the colon, which leads to a decrease in the production of secondary bile acids such as deoxycholate, and subsequently, less bile acids are absorbed [114, 115]. Increasing the absorption of deoxycholate can stimulate biliary cholesterol saturation [16, 116]. Significant reverse associations were observed between odds of gallstone disease and each category of dietary fiber intake. The relationship between dietary fiber intake and the risk of gallstones was more prominent in overweight and obese subjects than in subjects with a normal body mass index [117]. It appears that the fiber effect is multifaceted and potentially extremely complex in its influence on lipoproteins, bile acids, bile lipids, and intestinal sterols, including metabolism by the large bowel flora; therefore, an independent effect of fiber on gallbladder disease needs to be carefully analyzed.

Healthy nutrition recommends eating foods rich in fiber such as fruits and vegetables (FVs). Many constituents of fruits and vegetables may reduce the risk for gallstones, but prospective data relating fruit and vegetable intake to gallstone disease are sparse. An identification of the relationship between vegetables and fruits consumption and gallstone disease may provide the opportunity to reduce occurrence of gallstone disease. Higher consumption of fruit and vegetables is recommended as part of a healthy diet, which might be protective against gallstone disease [118, 119]. However, no unequivocal correlation of FVs consumption with the risk of developing gallstones has been identified. The protective role of FVs consumption on decreasing gallstone risk has been reported in several studies, [110, 120–123], whereas other studies could not confirm an association [124–127]. In addition, FVs consumption has been revealed to be negatively correlated with gallstone risk in other researches [125, 128]. Moreover, a linear dose-response correlation indicated that gallstone risk was reduced by 3 and 4% for every 200g per day increment in FVs consumption, respectively [129]. This inverse association can be explained because a higher FVs consumption increases dietary fiber, which shortens the intestinal transit [114], and dietary fiber has been inversely related to gallstone disease risk [130]. Experimental researches indicated that dietary fiber might decrease both total and LDL cholesterol by increasing bile acid excretion and decreasing hepatic synthesis of cholesterol [131]. In addition, higher FVs consumption possibly reduces fat intake [114]. A recent systematic review and meta-analysis has supported the thesis of a high consumption of FVs as a healthy diet and its recommendation for people to decrease the risk of symptomatic gallstone disease requiring cholecystectomy [129].

2.7 Vitamins and minerals intake

Clinical and experimental data in guinea pigs reported in the 1970s suggested a potential protective effect of vitamin C on the formation of gallstones [132, 133]. Furthermore, animal experiments have shown that animals deficient in vitamin C more frequently develop gallstones [134, 135]. An increased development of gallstones in subjects with vitamin C deficiency might also exist in humans [136]. While a report showed that short-term subclinical vitamin C deficiency in five healthy volunteers did not increase the lithogenic potential of gallbladder bile as it did in guinea pigs fed a high cholesterol diet, another study described changes in the bile salt composition and biliary phospholipid levels of vitamin C treated cholesterol gallstone patients and also found support for the notion that vitamin C supplementation might influence the conditions of cholesterol gallstone formation in humans [137, 138]. In humans, observational studies have also suggested an inverse association between vitamin C intake and gallstone disease [24, 121, 139, 140]. Another study evaluated the potential association of regular vitamin C supplement use on gallstone prevalence, as assessed by ultrasonography and patient's history, in a cross-sectional survey of randomly selected subjects from the general population. They concluded that gallstone prevalence was half in subjects with regular intake of vitamin C (powder, tablets or capsules) as compared to those not taking the vitamin [141]. A group of patients with cholelithiasis and elective surgery were treated with vitamin C (2 g per day for 2 weeks) orally for 2 weeks before surgery. Vitamin C supplementation did not change significantly plasma lipids and bile lipid concentrations, but in supplemented patients, significant reductions in biliary vesicular cholesterol content and biliary vesicular cholesterol/phospholipid ratio were observed [142]. Summing up, a vitamin C deficiency appears to promote gallstone formation, whereas a vitamin C supplement prevents lithogenesis. Vitamin C modulates the hepatic and biliary pathways of cholesterol homeostasis by promoting the conversion of cholesterol into bile acids through liver 7α-hydroxylation, by prolongation of the crystallization time [138] due to qualitative changes in the bile acid composition, and by a decrease in the cholesterol content of the thermodynamically unstable vesicles in the bile [142].

There are few studies on other vitamins and minerals. Calcium intake was inversely associated with gallstone incidence [24, 41, 143], but others found no association [44, 144]. Calcium may alter the composition of bile by preventing the reabsorption of secondary bile acids in the colon, thus reducing the deoxycholate and cholesterol content of the bile [145].

Animals receiving an iron-deficient diet were more likely to have cholesterol crystals in their bile than those on the control diet, suggesting that a low-iron diet may increase the risk of forming gallstones [146]. Some studies have reported associations with vitamin E [144], folate, or magnesium deficiency [147], but they are few and inconclusive [24, 144].

2.8 Coffee consumption

Metabolic studies suggest that coffee intake may influence gallstone formation [148–153]. Many studies indicate a potential protective effect of caffeine on gallstone formation [154–159]. On the other hand, other studies are not so clear in showing this effect [105, 160, 161], showing contradictory results. The effect is mainly mediated by the decreased hepatic synthesis and secretion of cholesterol [151, 153] and a positive effect on gallbladder motility [148, 150] and intestinal [162]. An inverse association between coffee consumption and risk of cholecystectomy in women who were premenopausal or used hormone replacement therapy but not in other women or in men was observed [163]. This indicates that the observed association between coffee consumption and cholecystectomy depended on the presence of female sex hormones. In view of the heterogeneous findings from other studies, the true nature of this association is yet to be established.

2.9 Alcohol consumption

Notwithstanding that alcohol consumption is a known risk factor for many chronic diseases and malignancies [164–166], there have been many clinical epidemiological studies regarding the negative correlation between alcohol consumption and gallstone disease risk. There were two published meta-analyses regarding the correlation between alcohol consumption and gallstone development risk [167, 168]. One meta-analysis found no significant correlation between alcohol consumption and incidental gallstone risks [167]. Another meta-analysis showed a statistically significant, inverse relationship between the highest and lowest consumption categories (RR, 0.62; 95% CI, 0.49 to 0.78), whose pooled risk reduction was larger than that of the overall drinking data relative to nondrinking or to the lowest category in this meta-analysis [168]. Other study discovered a trend of linear decline in gallstone disease risk according to an increase in alcohol consumption and a weakened linear trend between 28 and 40 g/day compared to that of under 28 g/day in the overall and case-control studies but not in the cohort studies [169]. Later studies demonstrated an inverse relation between consumption of different alcoholic beverages (wine, beer, liquors) and the risk of cholecystectomy [170], while a protective effect of small doses of alcohol (particularly in men) was documented in the cohort from the European Prospective Investigation into Cancer-Norfolk (EPIC-Norfolk) [171]. However, the topic is controversial in many respects: not all studies have confirmed the protective effect of alcohol on gallstone disease [105, 172]. Such general pathophysiological effect of alcohol on biliary function needs clinical confirmation. Alcohol inhibits the cholesteryl ester transfer protein (CETP)-mediated conversion of HDL into low-density lipoprotein (LDL)-cholesterol [173]. This step is followed by increased HDL cholesterol concentrations, which are inversely correlated with biliary cholesterol saturation [174, 175]. Small doses of alcohol also stimulate gallbladder contractility through increased cholecystokinin release [176, 177]. In general, the results of the effect of alcohol on gallstone formation are inconsistent, and it appears that the metabolic status of the host may be an important variable.

2.10 Nicotine and lithogenic diet

Some research has shown an influence of smoking on the development of gallstones [178, 179]. On the other hand, several studies suggest that smoking is not a risk factor for gallstones and even has the opposite effect [180, 181]. Compared with nonsmokers, older smokers who smoke for most of their lives have a lower risk of gallstone disease [182]. Megalin and cubilin proteins are expressed in gallbladder epithelial cells but not in hepatocytes. Dysregulation of megalin and cubilin at the mRNA and protein levels has been found in either humans or mice with gallstones [183, 184]. It was shown that bile acids can regulate the expression of megalin and cubilin, an effect that appeared to be mediated by the bile acid nuclear hormone receptor farnesoid X receptor (FXR) [185]. FXR can regulate the synthesis of bile acids in a tissue-specific manner, regulating bile acid reabsorption, maintaining bile acid cycle homeostasis, and reducing cholesterol and fat production [186]. In animals treated with a lithogenic diet, it was found that nicotine did not prevent cholesterol gallstone formation, but decreased biliary cholesterol secretion, retarding phase transition of cholesterol and that this is likely due to nicotine changing the expression of FXR/megalin pathway [187]. Despite unlikely therapeutic applications, nicotine might have potential beneficial effects for anti-lithogenic activity. However, further assessment of the direct effect of megalin and cubilin regulated by nicotine on gallstone formation is required.

3. Diet after cholecystectomy

Previous studies show that long-term abdominal symptoms are present in up to 40% of patients after laparoscopic cholecystectomy [188–190], which are summarized as "postcholecystectomy síndrome". It is thought that the symptoms are not caused by, but are exacerbated by, the cholecystectomy. Symptoms may include upset stomach, nausea, vomiting, gas, bloating, diarrea, or persistent pain in the upper right abdomen. The absence of the gallbladder after a cholecystectomy was reported to cause rapid enterohepatic recycling, an increase in the secretion and a decrease in the reabsorption of bile acid, and a shortened colonic transit time [191, 192]. Some patients who underwent cholecystectomy experienced diarrhea, which could be associated with the malabsorption of bile acid [193]. In addition, patients may experience symptoms of gastritis secondary to duodenogastric reflux of bile acids [191]. These abdominal symptoms suggest a relationship between cholecystectomic symptoms and diet, although the details of this association remain unclear.

There is not a standard guideline for medical nutrition theraphy postcholecystectomy. Many studies have focused on the relationship between a high-fat diet and postcholecystectomic syndromes [194–197]. A high-fat diet could be associated with postcholecystectomic diarrhea, due to the changes in bile acid metabolism. However, more recent research has not found a significant association between the intake of fat and the risk for postcholecystectomic syndromes [198, 199]. A low-fat diet does not seem to have an influence on the improvement of symptoms after cholecystectomy [199]. Despite this, it is recommended that fat intake should be limited for several months to allow the liver to compensate for the gallbladder's absence, should be introduced gradually, and excessive amounts at any one meal should be avoided [200]. Eggs could be a source of animal protein and cholesterol, which were also positively associated with the risk of postcholecystectomic syndromes [198]. Intake of protein had been reported to slow gastric emptying in healthy volunteers [201], and dietary cholesterol increased fecal excretion of bile acids in rats [202]. Malabsorption of bile acids has been shown to cause postcholecystectomic diarrhea [193, 203], since the absence of a gallbladder caused more rapid enterohepatic recycling of bile acids, increased bile acid secretion [193], and shortened colonic transit times [192]. The aforementioned studies suggested that excretion and malabsorption of bile acids could be exacerbated by cholesterol intake in patients with cholecystectomies. On the other hand, an increased fiber intake will help normalize bowel movements. It is recommended to increase fiber intake slowly, over several weeks [198, 200]. It has been suggested that adding soluble fiber to the diet will act as a sequestering agent and bind the bile in the stomach between meals to avoid gastritis [204]. In addition, symptomatic patients consumed more bread-based breakfast foods, while asymptomatic patients consumed more rice [198]. Another study found that the risk of nonalcoholic fatty liver disease (NAFLD) was negatively associated with a healthy dietary pattern of consuming whole grains, legumes, vegetables, fish, and fruit and with an erythrocyte level of n-3 polyunsaturated fatty acids rich in fish [205].

Therefore, it is important for patients who have undergone cholecystectomy to maintain a healthy diet that is rich in whole grains, legumes, vegetables, fish, and fruit and low in animal protein, cholesterol, and eggs. Additionally, it is recommended to avoid refined grains, meat, processed meat, and fried foods, which were positively associated with the risk of NAFLD [205]. However, each patient's dietary needs may vary, and it is recommended to consult with a healthcare professional or a registered dietitian for personalized dietary recommendations.

4. Conclusion

The high prevalence of cholesterol gallstones, the availability of new information about pathogenesis, and the relevant health costs due to the management of cholelithiasis in both children and adults contribute to a growing interest in this disease. Gallstone formation is multifactorial, resulting from an intricate interaction between multiple genetic, environmental, and lifestyle determinants. Cholelithiasis appears as the expression of systemic unbalances that, besides the classic therapeutic approaches to patients with clinical evidence of symptomatic disease or complications (mainly surgery), could be managed with tools oriented to primary prevention such as diet and lifestyle changes, which could imply a reduction in both prevalence and health costs. A major intervention in the general population should include lifestyle change, including dietary models able to possibly reduce the risk of gallstones mainly acting on lipid metabolism and metabolic pathways leading to gallstone formation. The risk of developing gallstones appears to increase with some dietary factors such as an increased of energy intake, low dietary fiber content, high refined sugar intake, and high fructose and fat intake and, on the other hand, to decrease with others like olive oil consumption (ω-3 fatty acids), high intake of monounsaturated fats and fiber, vegetables and fruits, vitamin C supplementation, nut consumption, dietary magnesium-calcium-iron supplementation, and moderate alcohol consumption (**Figure 1**) [1, 13, 15].

The complex and variable interactions of such pathogenic factors contributing to cholesterol cholelithiasis require a comprehensive discussion to correctly address the management of the disease. Studies that defined specific population with the consideration of multidimensional factors should be employed during the screening of populations with cholelithiasis. A better understanding of the role of diet in the formation of gallstones can provide resources and education to those patients who have been diagnosed with symptomatic gallstones and can also aid in the prevention and therapy of cholelithiasis.

Acknowledgements

- This work was partially supported by DINREG 12/2017 project (Direccion Investigacion, Universidad Catolica de la Santisima Concepcion).

- The graphic work of the Unit of Graphic Support (UAD) of Medicine Faculty, Universidad Catolica de la Santisima Concepcion, is appreciated.

Author details

Reginald del Pozo
Universidad Catolica de la Santisima Concepcion, Concepcion, Chile

*Address all correspondence to: rpozo@ucsc.cl

References

[1] Pak M, Lindseth G. Risk factors for cholelithiasis. Gastroenterology Nursing. 2016;**39**(4):297-309. DOI: 10.1097/SGA.0000000000000235

[2] Lammert F, Sauerbruch T. Mechanisms of disease: The genetic epidemiology of gallbladder stones. Nature Clinical Practice. Gastroenterology & Hepatology. 2005;**2**(9):423-433

[3] Dowling RH. Review: Pathogenesis of gallstones. Alimentary Pharmacology & Therapeutics. 2000;**14**(Suppl 2): 39-47. DOI: 10.1046/j.1365-2036.2000.014s2039.x

[4] Lammert F, Gurusamy Ko CW, Miquel JF, Mendez-Sanchez N, Portincasa P, van Erpecum KJ, et al. Gallstones. Nature Reviews. Disease Primers. 2016;**2**:16024. DOI: 10.1038/nrdp.2016.24

[5] Hofmann AF. Bile acid secretion, bile flow and biliary lipid secretion in humans. Hepatology. 1990;**12**(3 Pt 2):17S-22S discussion 22S-25S

[6] Portincasa P, Moschetta A, Palasciano G. Cholesterol gallstone disease. Lancet. 2006;**368**(9531):230-239. DOI: 10.1016/S0140-6736(06)69044-2

[7] Méndez-Sánchez N, Cárdenas-Vásquez R, Ponciano-Rodríguez G, et al. Pathophysiology of cholesterol gallstone disease. Archives of Medical Research. 1996;**27**(4):433-441

[8] Holzbach RT. Current concepts of cholesterol transport and crystal formation in human bile. Hepatology. 1990;**12**(3 Pt 2):26S-31S discussion 31S-32S

[9] Lagarriga Attias J, Mendez-Sanchez N, Chiprut Obadia RS, Cohen YJ. Experimental cholelithiasis in animals. Revista de Gastroenterología de México. 1978;**43**(3):147-161

[10] Cuevas A, Miquel JF, Reyes MS, Zanlungo S, Nervi F. Diet as a risk factor for cholesterol gallstone disease. Journal of the American College of Nutrition. 2004;**23**(3):187-196. DOI: 10.1080/07315724.2004.10719360

[11] Paumgartner G, Sauerbruch T. Gallstones: Pathogenesis. Lancet. 1991;**338**(8775):1117-1121. DOI: 10.1016/0140-6736(91)91972-w

[12] Stokes CS, Lammert F. Excess body weight and gallstone disease. Visceral Medicine. 2021;**37**(4):254-260. DOI: 10.1159/000516418

[13] Di Ciaula A, Portincasa P. Recent advances in understanding and managing cholesterol gallstones. F1000Res. 2018;**7**:F1000. DOI: 10.12688/f1000research.15505.1 eCollection 2018

[14] Mendez-Sanchez N, Bahena-Aponte J, Chavez-Tapia NC, Motola-Kuba D, Sanchez-Lara K, Ponciano-Rodriguez G, et al. Strong association between gallstones and cardiovascular disease. The American Journal of Gastroenterology. 2005;**100**(4):827-830. DOI: 10.1111/j.1572-0241.2005.41214.x

[15] Di Ciaula A, Garruti G, Frühbeck G, De Angelis M, de Bari O, Wang D, et al. The role of diet in the pathogenesis of cholesterol gallstones. Current Medicinal Chemistry. 2019;**26**(19):3620-3638. DOI: 10.2174/09298673246661 70530080636

[16] Hayes KC, Livingston A, Trautwein EA. Dietary impact on

biliary lipids and gallstones. Annual Review of Nutrition. 1992;**12**:299-326. DOI: 10.1146/annurev.nu.12.070192.001503

[17] Apstein MD, Carey MC. Pathogenesis of cholesterol gallstones: A parsimonious hypothesis. European Journal of Clinical Investigation. 1996;**26**(5):343-352. DOI: 10.1046/j.1365-2362.1996.148287.x

[18] Maclure KM, Hayes KC, Colditz GA, Stampfer MJ, Speizer FE, Willett WC. Weight, diet, and the risk of symptomatic gallstones in middle-aged women. The New England Journal of Medicine. 1989;**321**(9):563-569. DOI: 10.1056/NEJM198908313210902

[19] Bennion LJ, Grundy SM. Risk factors for the development of cholelithiasis in man. The New England Journal of Medicine. 1978;**299**(22):1221-1227. DOI: 10.1056/NEJM197811302992205

[20] Liu T, Siyin ST, Tao N, Duan N, Xu G, Li W, et al. Relationship between high-sensitivity C reactive protein and the risk of gallstone disease: Results from the Kailuan cohort study. BMJ Open. 2020;**10**(9):e035880. DOI: 10.1136/bmjopen-2019-035880

[21] Kwaifa IK, Bahari H, Yong YK, Noor SM. Endothelial dysfunction in obesity-induced inflammation: Molecular mechanisms and clinical implications. Biomolecules. 2020;**10**(2):291. DOI: 10.3390/biom10020291

[22] Cozma A, Orasan O, Sampelean D, Fodor A, Vlad C, Negrean V, et al. Endothelial dysfunction in metabolic sindrome. Romanian Journal of Internal Medicine. 2009;**47**(2):133-140

[23] Caroli-Bosc FX, Deveau C, Peten EP, Delabre P, Zanaldi H, Hebuterne X, et al. Cholelithiasis and dietary risk factors: An epidemiologic investigation in Vidauban, Southeast France. General Practitioner's group of Vidauban. Digestive Diseases and Sciences. 1998;**43**(9):2131-2137. DOI: 10.1023/a:1018879819301

[24] Ortega RM, Fernandez-Azuela M, Encinas Sotillos A, Andres P, Lopez-Sobaler AM. Differences in diet and food habits between patients with gallstones and controls. Journal of the American College of Nutrition. 1997;**16**(1):88-95. DOI: 10.1080/07315724.1997.10718655

[25] Stender S, Nordestgaard BG, Tybjaerg-Hansen A. Elevated body mass index as a causal risk factor for symptomatic gallstone disease: A Mendelian randomization study. Hepatology. 2013;**58**(6):2133-2141. DOI: 10.1002/hep.26563

[26] Haffner SM, Diehl AK, Stern MP, Hazuda HP. Central adiposity and gallbladder disease in Mexican Americans. American Journal of Epidemiology. 1989;**129**(3):587-595. DOI: 10.1093/oxfordjournals.aje.a115171

[27] Wang DQH, Neuschwander-Tetri BA, Portincasa P. The Biliary System. 1st ed. Princeton, New Jersey: Morgan & Claypool Life Sciences; 2012. pp. 1-146

[28] Stahlberg D, Rudling M, Angelin B, Bjorkhem I, Forsell P, Nilsell K, et al. Hepatic cholesterol metabolism in human obesity. Hepatology. 1997;**25**(6):1447-1450. DOI: 10.1002/hep.510250623

[29] Di Ciaula A, Wang DQ, Portincasa P. Gallbladder and gastric motility in obese newborns, preadolescents and adults. Journal of Gastroenterology and Hepatology. 2012;**27**(8):1298-1305. DOI: 10.1111/j.1440-1746.2012.07149.x

[30] Mathus-Vliegen EM, Van Ierland-Van Leeuwen ML,

Terpstra A. Determinants of gallbladder kinetics in obesity. Digestive Diseases and Sciences 2004;**49**(1):9-16. DOI: 10.1023/b:ddas.0000011595.39555.c0

[31] Tsai AG, Wadden TA. Systematic review: An evaluation of major comercial weight loss programs in the United States. Annals of Internal Medicine. 2005;**142**(1):56-66. DOI: 10.7326/0003-4819-142-1-200501040-00012

[32] Johansson K, Sundstrom J, Marcus C, Hemmingsson E, Neonius M. Risk of symptomatic gallstones and cholecystectomy after a very-low-calorie diet or low-calorie diet in a comercial weight los programm: 1-year matched cohort study. International Journal of Obesity. 2014;**38**(2):279-284. DOI: 10.1038/ijo.2013.83

[33] Li VK, Pulido N, Fajnwaks P, Szomstein S, Rosenthal R, Martinez-Duartz P. Predictors of gallstone formation after bariatric surgery: A multivariante analysis of risk factors comparing gastric bypass, gastric banding, and sleeve gastrectomy. Surgical Endoscopy. 2009;**23**(7):1640-1644. DOI: 10.1007/s00464-008-0204-6

[34] Broomfield PH, Chopra R, Sheinbaum RC, Bonorris GG, Silverman A, Schoenfield LJ, et al. Effects of Ursodeoxycholic acid and aspirin on the formation of Lithogenic bile and gallstones during loss of weight. The New England Journal of Medicine. 1988;**319**:1567-1572. DOI: 10.1056/NEJM198812153192403

[35] Jang S, Fang S, Kim KP, Ko Y, Kim H, Oh J, et al. Combination treatment with n-3 polyunsaturated fatty acids and ursodeoxycholic acid dissolves cholesterol gallstones in mice. Scientific Reports. 2019;**9**(1):12740. DOI: 10.1038/s41598-019-49095-z

[36] Jüngst D, Brenner G, Pratschke E, Paumgartner G. Low-dose ursodeoxycholic acid prolongs cholesterol nucleation time in gallbladder bile of patients with cholesterol gallstones. Journal of Hepatology. 1989;**8**(1):1-6. DOI: 10.1016/0168-8278(89)90154-2

[37] Jüngst C, Sreejayan N, Zündt B, Müller I, Spelsberg FW, Hüttl TP, et al. Ursodeoxycholic acid reduces lipid peroxidation and mucin secretagogue activity in gallbladder bile of patients with cholesterol gallstones. European Journal of Clinical Investigation. 2008;**38**(9):634-639. DOI: 10.1111/j.1365-2362.2008.01995.x

[38] Gutt C, Schläfer S, Lammert F. The treatment of gallstone disease. Deutsches Ärzteblatt International. 2020;**117**(9):148-158. DOI: 10.3238/arztebl.2020.0148

[39] Su PY, Hsu YC, Cheng YF, Kor CT, Su WW. Strong association between metabolically abnormal obesity and gallstone disease in adults under 50 years. BMC Gastroenterology. 2019;**19**(1):117. DOI: 10.1186/s12876-019-1032-y

[40] Jorgensen T, Jorgensen LM. Gallstones and diet in a Danish population. Scandinavian Journal of Gastroenterology. 1989;**24**(7):821-826. DOI: 10.3109/00365528909089221

[41] Moerman CJ, Smeets FW, Kromhout D. Dietary risk factors for clinically diagnosed gallstones in middle-aged men. A 25-year follow-up study. Annals of Epidemiology. 1994;**4**(3):248-254. DOI: 10.1016/1047-2797(94)90104-x

[42] Attili AF, Scafato E, Marchioli R, Marfisi RM, Festi D. Diet and gallstones in Italy: Cross-sectional MICOL results. Hepatology. 1998;**27**(6):1492-1498. DOI: 10.1002/hep.510270605

[43] Yago MD, Gonzalez V, Serrano P, et al. Effect of the type of dietary fat on biliary lipid composition and bile lithogenicity in humans with cholesterol gallstone disease. Nutrition. 2005;**21**(3):339-347. DOI: 10.1016/j.nut.2004.06.028

[44] Sichierei R, Everhart JE, Roth H. A propspective study of hospitalization with gallstone disease among women: Role of dietary factors, fasting period, and dieting. American Journal of Public Health. 1991;**81**(7):880-884. DOI: 10.2105/ajph.81.7.880

[45] Misciagna G, Centonze S, Leoci C, Guerra V, Cisternino AM, Ceo R, et al. Diet, physical activity, and gallstones: A population-based, case-control study in southern Italy. The American Journal of Clinical Nutrition. 1999;**69**(1):120-126. DOI: 10.1093/ajcn/69.1.120

[46] del Pozo R, Mardones L, Villagran M, Muñoz K, Roa S, Rozas F, et al. Effect of a high-fat diet on cholesterol gallstone formation. Revista Médica de Chile. 2017;**145**(9):1099-1105

[47] Tsai CJ, Leitzmann MF, Willett WC, Giovannucci EL. Long-term intake of trans-fatty acids and risk of gallstone disease in men. Archives of Internal Medicine. 2005;**165**(9):1011-1015. DOI: 10.1001/archinte.165.9.1011

[48] Tsai CJ, Leitzmann MF, Willett WC, Giovannucci EL. The effect of long-term intake of cis unsaturated fats on the risk for gallstone disease in men: A prospective cohort study. Annals of Internal Medicine. 2004;**141**(7):514-522. DOI: 10.7326/0003-4819-141-7-200410050-00007

[49] Jonnalagadda SS, Trautwein EA, Hayes KC. Dietary fats rich in saturated fatty acids (12:0, 14:0, and 16:0) enhance gallstone formation relative to monounsaturated fat (18:1) in cholesterol-fed hamsters. Lipids. 1995;**30**(5):415-424. DOI: 10.1007/BF02536299

[50] Tandon RK, Saraya A, Paul S, Kapur BM. Dietary habits of gallstone patients in northern India. Journal of Clinical Gastroenterology. 1996;**22**(1):23-27. DOI: 10.1097/00004836-199601000-00007

[51] Schlierf G, Nikolaus T, Stichl A, et al. The effect of lipid level lowering diets on bile lipids and plasma lipoproteins in normal persons. Schweizerische Medizinische Wochenschrift. 1979;**109**(45):1743-1747

[52] Soo-Min C, Jin-A P, Dong-Soon K, Zhang D, Yi H, Hee-Jung C, et al. Effect of eicosapentaenoic acid on cholesterol gallstone formation in C57BL/6J mice. Molecular Medicine Reports. 2015;**11**(1):362-366. DOI: 10.3892/mmr.2014.2687

[53] Jonkers IJ, Smelt AH, Ledeboer M, Hollum ME, Biemond I, Kuipers F, et al. Gallbladder dysmotility: A risk factor for gallstone formation in hypertriglyceridaemia and reversal on triglyceride lowering therapy by bezafibrate and fish oil. Gut. 2003;**52**(1):109-115. DOI: 10.1136/gut.52.1.109

[54] Magnuson TH, Lillemoe KD, High RC, Pitt HA. Dietary fish oil inhibits cholesterol monohydrate crystal nucleation and gallstone formation in the prairie dog. Surgery. 1995;**118**(3):517-523. DOI: 10.1016/s0039-6060(05)80368-x

[55] Berr F, Holl J, Jüngst D, Fischer S, Richter WO, Seifferth B, et al. Dietary n-3 polyunsaturated fatty acids decrease biliary cholesterol saturation in gallstone disease. Hepatology. 1992;**16**(4):960-967. DOI: 10.1002/hep.1840160418

[56] Mendez-Sanchez N, Gonzalez V, Aguayo P, Sanchez JM, Tanimoto MA, Elizondo J, et al. Fish oil (n-3) polyunsaturated fatty acids beneficially affect biliary cholesterol nucleation time in obese women losing weight. The Journal of Nutrition. 2001;**131**(9):2300-2303. DOI: 10.1093/jn/131.9.2300

[57] Booker ML, Scott TE, LaMorte WW. Effects of dietary fish oil on biliary phospholipids and prostaglandin synthesis in the cholesterol-fed prairie dog. Lipids. 1990;**25**(1):27-32. DOI: 10.1007/BF02562424

[58] Almario RU, Vonghavaravat V, Wong R, Kasim-Karakas SE. Effects of walnut consumption on plasma fatty acids and lipoproteins in combined hyperlipidemia. American Journal of Clinical Nutrition. 2001;**74**(1):72-79. DOI: 10.1093/ajcn/74.1.72

[59] Tsai CJ, Leitzmann MF, Hu FB, Willett WC, Giovannucci EL. A prospective cohort study of nut consumption and the risk of gallstone disease. American Journal of Epidemiology. 2004;**160**(1):961-968. DOI: 10.1093/aje/kwh302

[60] Kris-Etherton PM, Zhao G, Binkoski AE, Coval SE, Etherton TD. The effects of nuts on coronary heart disease risk. Nutrition Reviews. 2001;**59**:103-111. DOI: 10.1111/j.1753-4887.2001.tb06996.x

[61] Rajaram S, Burke K, Connell B, Myint T, Sabate J. A monounsaturated fatty acid-rich pecan-enriched diet favorably laters the serum lipid profile of healthy men and women. Journal of Nutrition. 2001;**131**:2275-2279. DOI: 10.1093/jn/131.9.2275

[62] Lee DW, Gilmore CJ, Bonorris G, Cohen H, Marks JW, et al. Effect of dietary cholesterol on biliary lipids in patients with gallstones and normal subjects and persons with gallstones. The American Journal of Clinical Nutrition. 1985;**42**(3):414-420. DOI: 10.1093/ajcn/42.3.414

[63] DenBesten L, Connor WE, Bell S. The effect of dietary cholesterol on the composition of human bile. Surgery. 1973;**73**(2):266-273

[64] Tepperman J, Caldwell FT, Tepperman HM. Induction of gallstones in mice by feeding a cholesterol-cholic acid containing diet. The American Journal of Physiology. 1964;**206**:628-634. DOI: 10.1152/ajplegacy.1964.206.3.628

[65] Hayes KC, Khosla P, Pronczuk A. Diet-induced type IV-like hyperlipidemia and increased body weight are associated with cholesterol gallstones in hamsters. Lipids. 1991;**26**(9):729-735. DOI: 10.1007/BF02535622

[66] Mitchell JC, Loan GM, Stone BG, Duane WC. Effects of lovastatin on biliary lipid secretion and bile acid metabolism in humans. Journal of Lipid Research. 1991;**32**(1):71-78

[67] Ho KJ. Comparative studies on the effect of cholesterol feeding on biliary composition. The American Journal of Clinical Nutrition. 1976;**29**(7):698-704. DOI: 10.1093/ajcn/29.7.698

[68] Méndez-Sánchez N, Zamora-Valdés D, Chávez-Tapia NC, Uribe M. Role of diet in cholesterol gallstone formation. Clinica Chimica Acta. 2007;**376**(1-2):1-8. DOI: 10.1016/j.cca.2006.08.036

[69] Goswami SK, Frey CF. Effect of beta-sitosterol on cholesterol-cholic acid-induced gallstone formation in mice. The American Journal of Gastroenterology. 1976;**65**(4):305-310

[70] Shen W, Wang Y, Shao W, Wang Q, Jiang Z, Hu H. Dietary plant sterols prevented cholesterol gallstone formation in mice. Food & Function. 2021;**12**(23):11829-11837. DOI: 10.1039/d1fo02695j

[71] Ulloa N, Nervi F. Mechanism and kinetic characteristics of the uncoupling by plant steroids of biliary cholesterol from bile salt output. Biochimica et Biophysica Acta. 1985;**837**(2):181-189. DOI: 10.1016/0005-2760(85)90241-3

[72] Nervi F, Covarrubias C, Bravo P, Velasco N, Ulloa N, Cruz F, et al. Influence of legume intake on biliary lipids and cholesterol saturation in young Chilean men. Gastroenterology. 1989;**96**(3):825-830

[73] Duane WC. Effects of legume consumption on serum cholesterol, biliary lipids, and sterol metabolism in humans. Journal of Lipid Research. 1997;**38**(6):1120-1128

[74] Scragg RK, McMichael AJ, Baghurst PA. Diet, alcohol, and relative weight in gallstone disease: A case-control study. British Medical Journal (Clinical Research Ed.). 1984;**288**(6424):1113-1119. DOI: 10.1136/bmj.288.6424.1113

[75] Diehl AK, Haffner SM, Knapp JA, Hazuda HP, Stern MP. Dietary intake and the prevalence of gallbladder disease in Mexican Americans. Gastroenterology. 1989;**97**(6):1527-1533. DOI: 10.1016/0016-5085(89)90399-5

[76] Thornton JR, Emmet P, Heaton KW. Diet and gallstones: Effect of refined and unrefined carbohydrate diets on bile cholesterol saturation and bile acid metabolism. Gut. 1983;**24**(1):2-6. DOI: 10.1136/gut.24.1.2

[77] Arbeitsgemeinschaft der Wissenschaftlichen Medizinischen Fachgesellschaften (AWMF). Interdisziplinäre Leitlinie der Qualität S3 zur Prävention und Therapie der Adipositas-Gesellschaft. Martinsried: AWMF; 2014

[78] Tsai CJ, Leitzmann MF, Willett WC, Giovannucci EL. Glycemic load, glycemic index, and carbohydrate intake in relation to risk of cholecystectomy in women. Gastroenterology. 2005;**129**(1):105-112. DOI: 10.1053/j.gastro.2005.05.016

[79] Wong AC, Ko CW. Carbohydrate intake as a risk factor for biliary sludge and stones during pregnancy. Journal of Clinical Gastroenterology. 2013;**47**(8):700-705. DOI: 10.1097/MCG.0b013e318286fdb0

[80] Mathur A, Megan M, Al-Azzawi HH, Lu D, Swartz-Basile DA, Nakeeb A, et al. High dietary carbohydrates decrease gallbladder volume and enhance cholesterol crystal formation. Surgery. 2007;**141**(5):654-659. DOI: 10.1016/j.surg.2006.11.008

[81] Vos MB, Kimmons JE, Gillespie C, Welsh J, Blanck HM. Dietary fructose consumption among US children and adults: The third National Health and nutrition examination survey. Medscape Journal of Medicine. 2008;**10**(7):160

[82] Softic S, Cohen DE, Kahn CR. Role of dietary fructose and hepatic de novo lipogenesis in fatty liver disease. Digestive Diseases and Sciences. 2016;**61**(5):1282-1293. DOI: 10.1007/s10620-016-4054-0

[83] Bizeau ME, Pagliassotti MJ. Hepatic adaptations to sucrose and fructose. Metabolism. 2005;**54**(9):1189-1201. DOI: 10.1016/j.metabol.2005.04.004

[84] Tappy L, Le KA. Metabolic effects of fructose and the worldwide increase in obesity. Physiological Reviews. 2010;**90**(1):23-46. DOI: 10.1152/physrev.00019.2009

[85] Jung S, Bae H, Song WS, Jang C. Dietary fructose and fructose-induced pathologies. Annual Review of Nutrition. 2022;**42**:45-66. DOI: 10.1146/annurev-nutr-062220-025831

[86] Faeh D, Minehira K, Schwarz JM, Periasamy R, Park S, Tappy L. Effect of fructose overfeeding and fish oil administration on hepatic *de novo* lipogenesis and insulin sensitivity in healthy men. Diabetes. 2005;**54**(7):1907-1913. DOI: 10.2337/diabetes.54.7.1907

[87] Dirlewanger M, Schneiter P, Jequier E, Tappy L. Effects of fructose on hepatic glucose metabolism in humans. American Journal of Physiology. Endocrinology and Metabolism. 2000;**279**:E907-E911

[88] Biddinger SB, Haas JT, Yu BB, Bezy O, Jing E, Zhang W, et al. Hepatic insulin resistance directly promotes formation of cholesterol gallstones. Nature Medicine. 2008;**14**(7):778-782. DOI: 10.1038/nm1785

[89] Tappy L, Le KA, Tran C, Paquot N. Fructose and metabolic diseases: New findings, new questions. Nutrition. 2010;**26**(11-12):1044-1049. DOI: 10.1016/j.nut.2010.02.014

[90] Tetri LH, Basaranoglu M, Brunt EM, Yerian LM, Neuschwander-Tetri BA. Severe NAFLD with hepatic necroinflammatory changes in mice fed trans fats and a high-fructose corn syrup equivalent. American Journal of Physiology. Gastrointestinal and Liver Physiology. 2008;**295**(5):G987-G995. DOI: 10.1152/ajpgi.90272.2008

[91] Stanhope KL, Bremer AA, Medici V, Nakajima K, Ito Y, Nakano T, et al. Consumption of fructose and high fructose corn syrup increase postprandial triglycerides, LDL-cholesterol, and apoliporotein-B in young men and women. The Journal of Clinical Endocrinology and Metabolism. 2011;**96**(10):E1596-E1605. DOI: 10.1210/jc.2011-1251

[92] Lim JS, Mietus-Snyder M, Valente A, Schwarz JM, Lustig RH. The role of fructose in the pathogenesis of NAFLD and the metabolic syndrome. Nature Reviews. Gastroenterology & Hepatology. 2010;**7**(5):251-264. DOI: 10.1038/nrgastro.2010.41

[93] Bonfrate L, Krawczyk M, Lembo A, Grattagliano I, Lammert F, Portincasa P. Effects of dietary education, followed by a tailored fructose-restricted diet in adults with fructose malabsorption. European Journal of Gastroenterology & Hepatology. 2015;**27**(7):785-796. DOI: 10.1097/MEG.0000000000000374

[94] Kahn R, Sievenpiper JL. Dietary sugar and body weight: Have we reached a crisis in the epidemic of obesity and diabetes?: We have, but the pox on sugar is overwrought and overworked. Diabetes Care. 2014;**37**(4):957-962. DOI: 10.2337/dc13-2506

[95] Tappy L, Mittendorfer B. Fructose toxicity: Is the science ready for public health actions? Current Opinion in Clinical Nutrition and Metabolic Care. 2012;**15**(4):357-361. DOI: 10.1097/MCO.0b013e328354727e

[96] del Pozo R, Mardones L, Villagran M, Muñoz K, Troncoso L, Mellado M, et al. Effect of various concentrations of dietary fructose on gallstone formation process in Balb/c mice. Nutricion Hospitalaria. 2023 (in press)

[97] Livesey G, Taylor R. Fructose consumption and consequences for glycation, plasma triglycerides and body weight: Meta-analyses and meta-regression models of intervention studies. The American Journal of Clinical Nutrition. 2008;**88**(5):1419-1437. DOI: 10.3945/ajcn.2007.25700

[98] Hou R, Panda C, Voruganti VS. Heterogeneity in metabolic responses to dietary fructose. Frontiers in Genetics. 2019;**10**:945. DOI: 10.3389/fgene.2019.00945

[99] Kritchevsky D, Klurfeld DM. Influence of vegetable protein on gallstone formation in hamsters. The American Journal of Clinical Nutrition. 1979;**32**:2174-2176. DOI: 10.1093/ajcn/32.11.2174

[100] Kritchevsky D, Klurfeld DM. Gallstone formation in hamsters: Effect of varying animal and vegetable protein levels. The American Journal of Clinical Nutrition. 1983;**37**(5):802-804. DOI: 10.1093/ajcn/37.5.802

[101] Mahfouz-Cercone S, Johnson JE, Liepa GU. Effect of dietary animal and vegetable protein on gallstone formation and biliary constituents in the hamster. Lipids. 1984;**19**(1):5-10. DOI: 10.1007/BF02534601

[102] Sullivan MA, Duffy A, Dimarco N, Liepa G. Effects of various dietary animal and vegetable proteins on serum and biliary lipids and on gallstone formation in the hamster. Lipids. 1985;**20**(1):1-6. DOI: 10.1007/BF02534354

[103] Tomotake H, Yamamoto N, Yanaka N, Ohinata H, Yamazaki R, Kayashita J, et al. High protein buckwheat flour suppresses hypercholesterolemia in rats and gallstone formation in mice by hypercholesterolemic diet and body fat in rats because of its low protein digestibility. Nutrition. 2006;**22**(2):166-173. DOI: 10.1016/j.nut.2005.01.012

[104] Catala I, Juste C, Boehler N, Ferezou J, Andre M, Riottot M, et al. Cholesterol crystallization in gall-bladder bile of pigs given cholesterol-beta-cyclodextrin-enriched diets with either casein or soyabean concentrate as protein sources. The British Journal of Nutrition. 2000;**83**(4):411-420

[105] Kratzer W, Kachele V, Mason RA, Muche R, Hay B, Wiesneth M, et al. Gallstone prevalence in relation to smoking, alcohol, coffee consumption, and nutrition. The Ulm gallstone study. Scandinavian Journal of Gastroenterology. 1997;**32**:953-958. DOI: 10.3109/00365529709011208

[106] Pixley F, Wilson D, McPherson K, Mann J. Effect of vegetarianism on development of gall stones in women. British Medical Journal (Clinical Research Ed.). 1985;**291**:11-12. DOI: 10.1136/bmj.291.6487.11

[107] Pradhan SB, Joshi MR, Vaidya A. Prevalence of different types of gallstone in the patients with cholelithiasis at Kathmandu medical college, Nepal. Kathmandu University Medical Journal (KUMJ). 2009;**7**(27):268-271

[108] Maclure KM, Hayes KC, Colditz GA, Stampfer MJ, Willett WC. Dietary predictors of symptom-associated gallstones in middle-aged women. The American Journal of Clinical Nutrition. 1990;**52**(5):916-922. DOI: 10.1093/ajcn/52.5.916

[109] Tsai CJ, Leitzmann MF, Willett WC, Giovannucci EL. Dietary protein and the risk of cholecystectomy in a cohort of US women: The nurses' health study. American Journal of Epidemiology. 2004;**160**(1):11-18. DOI: 10.1093/aje/kwh170

[110] Lander EM, Wertheim BC, Koch SM, Chen Z, Hsu CH, Thomson CA. Vegetable protein intake is associated with lower gallbladder disease risk: Findings from the Women's Health Initiative prospective cohort. Preventive Medicine. 2016;**88**:20-26. DOI: 10.1016/j.ypmed.2016.03.016

[111] Kameda H, Ishihara F, Shibata K, Tsukie E. Clinical and nutritional study on gallstone disease in Japan. Japanese Journal of Medicine. 1984;**23**(2):109-113. DOI: 10.2169/internalmedicine1962.23.109

[112] Scaggion GDS, Robbi R, Susanna S. Influence of dietary fibers in the genesis of cholesterol gallstone disease. Recenti Progressi in Medicina. 1988;**79**(6):246-248

[113] Schwesinger WH, Kurtin WE, Page CP, Stewart RM, Johnson R. Soluble dietary fiber protects against cholesterol gallstone formation. American Journal of Surgery. 1999;**177**(4):307-310. DOI: 10.1016/s0002-9610(99)00047-1

[114] Marcus S, Heaton K. Effects of a new, concentrated wheat fibre preparation on intestinal transit, deoxycholic acid metabolism and the composition of bile. Gut. 1986;**27**(8):893-900. DOI: 10.1136/gut.27.8.893

[115] Marcus SN, Heaton KW. Intestinal transit, deoxycholic acid and the cholesterol saturation of bile–three inter-related factors. Gut. 1986;**27**(5):550-558. DOI: 10.1136/gut.27.5.550

[116] Low-Beer TS. Nutrition and cholesterol gallstones. The Proceedings of the Nutrition Society. 1985;**44**(1):127-134. DOI: 10.1079/pns19850021

[117] Tehrani AN, Saadati S, Yari Z, Salehpour A, Sadeghi A, Daftari G, et al. Dietary fiber intake and risk of gallstone: A case-control study. BMC Gastroenterology. 2023;**23**(1):119. DOI: 10.1186/s12876-023-02752-0

[118] Waxman A. Prevention of chronic diseases: WHO global strategy on diet, physical activity and health. Food and Nutrition Bulletin. 2003;**24**(3):281-284. DOI: 10.1177/156482650302400306

[119] Lammert F, Acalovschi M, Ercolani G, et al. EASL clinical practice guidelines on the prevention, diagnosis and treatment of gallstones. Journal of Hepatology. 2016;**65**(1):146-181. DOI: 10.1016/j.jhep.2016.03.005

[120] Jessri M, Rashidkhani B. Dietary patterns and risk of gallbladder disease: A hospital-based case-control study in adult women. Journal of Health, Population, and Nutrition. 2015;**33**(1):39-49

[121] Tsai CJ, Leitzmann MF, Willett WC, et al. Fruit and vegetable consumption and risk of cholecystectomy in women. The American Journal of Medicine. 2006;**119**(9):760-767. DOI: 10.1016/j.amjmed.2006.02.040

[122] Bertola Compagnucci A, Perroud HA, Batallés SM, et al. A nested case-control study on dietary fat consumption and the risk for gallstone disease. Journal of Human Nutrition and Dietetics. 2016;**29**(3):338-344. DOI: 10.1111/jhn.12332

[123] Figueiredo JC, Haiman C, Porcel J, et al. Sex and ethnic/racial-specific risk factors for gallbladder disease. BMC Gastroenterology. 2017;**17**(1):153. DOI: 10.1186/s12876-017-0678-6

[124] Jayanthi V, Malathi S, Ramathilakam B, et al. Is vegetarianism a precipitating factor for gallstones in cirrhotics? Tropical Gastroenterology. 1998;**19**(1):21-23

[125] McConnell TJ, Appleby PN, Key TJ. Vegetarian diet as a risk factor for symptomatic gallstone disease. European Journal of Clinical Nutrition. 2017;**71**(6):731-735. DOI: 10.1038/ejcn.2016.252

[126] Rong Y, Chen L, Zhu T, et al. Egg consumption and risk of coronary heart disease and stroke: Dose-response meta-analysis of prospective cohort studies. BMJ. 2013;**346**:e8539. DOI: 10.1136/bmj.e8539

[127] Knobloch K, Yoon U, Vogt PM. Preferred reporting items for systematic reviews and meta-analyses (PRISMA) statement and publication bias. Journal of Cranio-Maxillo-Facial Surgery. 2011;**39**(2):91-92. DOI: 10.1016/j.jcms.2010.11.001

[128] Wang Y, Lu J, Wen N, Nie G, Peng D, Xiong X, et al. The role of diet and nutrition related indicators in biliary diseases: An umbrella review of systematic review and meta-analysis. Nutrition & Metabolism (London). 2022;**19**(1):51. DOI: 10.1186/s12986-022-00677-1

[129] Zhang JW, Xiong JP, Xu WY, Sang XT, Huang HC, Bian J, et al. Fruits and vegetables consumption and the risk of gallstone diasease: A systematic review and meta-analysis. Medicine (Baltimore). 2019;**98**(28):e16404. DOI: 10.1097/MD.0000000000016404

[130] Tsai CJ, Leitzmann MF, Willett WC, et al. Long-term intake of dietary fiber and decreased risk of cholecystectomy in women. The American Journal of Gastroenterology. 2004;**99**(7):1364-1370. DOI: 10.1111/j.1572-0241.2004.30153.x

[131] Hunninghake DB, Miller VT, Larosa JC, et al. Hypocholesterolemic effects of a dietary fiber supplement. The American Journal of Clinical Nutrition. 1994;**59**(5):1050-1054. DOI: 10.1093/ajcn/59.5.1050

[132] Ginter E. Cholesterol: Vitamin C controls its transformation to bile acids. Science. 1973;**179**(4074):702-704. DOI: 10.1126/science.179.4074.702

[133] Ginter E. Chenodeoxycholic acid, gallstones and vitamin C. The New England Journal of Medicine. 1976;**295**(22):1260-1261. DOI: 10.1056/NEJM197611252952218

[134] Jenkins SA. Hypovitaminosis C and cholelithiasis in Guinea pigs. Biochemical and Biophysical Research Communications. 1977;**77**(3):1030-1035. DOI: 10.1016/s0006-291x(77)80081-8

[135] Jenkins SA. Biliary lipids, bile acids and gallstone formation in hypovitaminotic C Guinea-pigs. The British Journal of Nutrition. 1978;**40**(2):317-322. DOI: 10.1079/bjn19780128

[136] Simon JA. Ascorbic acid and cholesterol gallstones. Medical Hypotheses. 1993;**40**(2):81-84. DOI: 10.1016/0306-9877(93)90132-a

[137] Duane WC, Hutton SW. Lack of effect of experimental ascorbic acid deficiency on bile acid metabolism, sterol balance, and biliary lipid composition in man. Journal of Lipid Research. 1983;**24**(9):1186-1195

[138] Gustafsson U, Wang FH, Axelson M, Kallner A, Sahlin S, Einarsson K. The effect of vitamin C in high doses on plasma and biliary lipid composition in patients with cholesterol gallstones: Prolongation of the nucleation time. European Journal of Clinical Investigation. 1997;**27**(5):387-391. DOI: 10.1046/j.1365-2362.1997.1240670.x

[139] Simon JA, Hudes ES. Serum ascorbic acid and other correlates of gallbladder disease among US adults. American Journal of Public Health. 1998;**88**(8):1208-1212. DOI: 10.2105/ajph.88.8.1208

[140] Simon JA, Hudes ES. Serum ascorbic acid and gallbladder disease prevalence among US adults: The third National Health and nutrition examination survey (NHANES III). Archives of Internal Medicine. 2000;**160**(7):931-936. DOI: 10.1001/archinte.160.7.931

[141] Walcher T, Haenle MM, Kron M, Hay B, Mason RA, Walcher D, et al. Vitamin C supplement use may protect against gallstones: An observational study on a randomly selected population. BMC Gastroenterology. 2009;**9**:74. DOI: 10.1186/1471-230X-9-74

[142] del Pozo R, Muñoz M, Dumas A, Tapia C, Muñoz K, Fuentes F, et al. Effects of vitamin C administration on cholesterol gallstone formation. Revista Médica de Chile. 2014;**142**(1):20-26. DOI: 10.4067/S0034-98872014000100004

[143] Williams CN, Johnston JL. Prevalence of gallstones and risk factors in Caucasian women in a rural Canadian community. Canadian Medical Association Journal. 1980;**122**(6):664-668

[144] Worthington HV, Hunt LP, McCloy RF, Maclennan I, Braganza JM. A pilot study of antioxidant intake in patients with cholesterol gallstones. Nutrition. 1997;**13**(2):118-127. DOI: 10.1016/s0899-9007(96)00385-1

[145] Van Der Meer R, Welberg JWM, Kuipers F, Kleibeuker JH, Mulder NH, Termont D, et al. Effects of supplemental dietary calcium on the intestinal association of calcium, phosphate, and bile acids. Gastroenterology. 1990;**99**(6):1653-1659. DOI: 10.1016/0016-5085(90)90471-c

[146] Johnston SM, Murray KP, Martin SA, Fox-Talbot K, Lipsett PA, Lillemoe KD, et al. Iron deficiency enhances cholesterol gallstone formation. Surgery. 1997;**122**(2):354-361; discussion 361-2. DOI: 10.1016/s0039-6060(97)90027-1

[147] Humphries S, Kushner H, Falkner B. Low dietary magnesium is associated with insulin resistance in a sample of young, nondiabetic black Americans. American Journal of Hypertension. 1999;**12**(8 Pt 1):747-756. DOI: 10.1016/s0895-7061(99)00041-2

[148] Douglas BR, Jansen JBMJ, Tham RTO, Lamers CBHW. Coffee stimulation of cholecystokinin release and gallbladder contraction in humans. The American Journal of Clinical Nutrition. 1990;**52**(3):553-556. DOI: 10.1093/ajcn/52.3.553

[149] Keiner F. The effect of coffee on gallbladder contraction. Die Medizinische Welt. 1965;**34**:1907-1912

[150] Magnuson TH, Zarkin BA, Lillemoe KD, May CA, Bastidas JA, Pitt HA. Caffeine inhibits gallbladder absorption. Current Surgery. 1989;**46**(6):477-479

[151] Lillemoe KD, Magnunson TH, High RC, Peoples GE, Pitt HA. Caffeine prevents cholesterol gallstone formation. Surgery. 1989;**106**(2):400-406 discussion 406-7

[152] Rustan AC, Halvorsen B, Huggett AC, Ranheim T, Drevon CA. Effect of coffee lipids (cafestol and kahweo) on regulation of cholesterol metabolism in HepG2 cells. Arteriosclerosis, Thrombosis, and

Vascular Biology. 1997;**17**(10):2140-2149. DOI: 10.1161/01.atv.17.10.2140

[153] Halvorsen B, Ranheim T, Nenseter MS, Huggets AC, Drevon CA. Effect of a coffee lipid (cafesol) on cholesterol metabolism in human skin fibroblast. Journal of Lipid Research. 1998;**39**(4):901-912

[154] La Vecchia C, Negri E, D'Avanzo B, Franceschi S, Boyle P. Risk factors for gallstone disease requiring surgery. International Journal of Epidemiology. 1991;**20**(1):209-215. DOI: 10.1093/ije/20.1.209

[155] Misciagna G, Leoci C, Guerra V, Chiloiro M, Elba S, Petruzzi J, et al. Epidemiology of cholelithiasis in southern Italy. Part II: Risk factors. European Journal of Gastroenterology & Hepatology. 1996;**8**(6):585-593. DOI: 10.1097/00042737-199606000-00017

[156] Leitzmann MF, Willett WC, Rimm EB, Stampfer MJ, Spiegelman D, Colditz GA, et al. A prospective study of coffee consumption and the risk of symptomatic gallstone disease in men. JAMA. 1999;**281**(22):2106-2112. DOI: 10.1001/jama.281.22.2106

[157] Ruhl CE, Everhart JE. Association of coffee consumption with gallbladder disease. American Journal of Epidemiology. 2000;**152**(11):1034-1038. DOI: 10.1093/aje/152.11.1034

[158] Leitzmann MF, Stampfer MJ, Willett WC, Spiegelman D, Colditz GA, Giovannucci EL. Coffee intake is associated with lower risk of symptomatic gallstone disease in women. Gastroenterology. 2002;**123**(6):1823-1830. DOI: 10.1053/gast.2002.37054

[159] Jorgensen T. Gall stones in a Danish population. Relation to weight, physical activity, smoking, coffee consumption, and diabetes mellitus. Gut. 1989;**30**(4):528-534. DOI: 10.1136/gut.30.4.528

[160] Walcher T, Haenle MM, Mason RA, Koenig W, Imhof A, Kratzer W, et al. The effect of alcohol, tobacco and caffeine consumption and vegetarian diet on gallstone prevalence. European Journal of Gastroenterology & Hepatology. 2010;**22**(11):1345-1351. DOI: 10.1097/MEG.0b013e32833efdb2

[161] Pastides H, Tzonou A, Trichopoulos D, Katsouyanni K, Trichopoulou A, Kefalogiannis N, et al. A case-control study of the relationship between smoking, diet, and gallbladder-disease. Archives of Internal Medicine. 1990;**150**(7):1409-1412

[162] Brown SR, Cann PA, Read NW. Effect of coffee on distal colon function. Gut. 1990;**31**(4):450-453. DOI: 10.1136/gut.31.4.450

[163] Nordenvall C, Oskarsson V, Wolk A. Inverse association between coffee consumption and risk of cholecystectomy in women but not in men. Clinical Gastroenterology and Hepatology. 2015;**13**(6):1096-1102.e1. DOI: 10.1016/j.cgh.2014.09.029

[164] Andreotti G, Liu E, Gao YT, et al. Medical history and the risk of biliary tract cancers in Shanghai, China: Implications for a role of inflammation. Cancer Causes & Control. 2011;**22**(9):1289-1296. DOI: 10.1007/s10552-011-9802-z

[165] Bagnardi V, Rota M, Botteri E, et al. Alcohol consumption and site-specific cancer risk: A comprehensive dose-response meta-analysis. British Journal of Cancer. 2015;**112**(3):580-593. DOI: 10.1038/bjc.2014.579

[166] Ahrens W, Timmer A, Vyberg M, et al. Risk factors for extrahepatic biliary tract carcinoma in men: Medical conditions and lifestyle: Results from a European multicentre case-control study. European Journal of Gastroenterology & Hepatology. 2007;**19**(8):623-630. DOI: 10.1097/01.meg.0000243876.79325.a1

[167] Shabanzadeh DM, Novovic S. Alcohol, smoking and benign hepatobiliary disease. Best Practice & Research. Clinical Gastroenterology. 2017;**31**(5):519-527. DOI: 10.1016/j.bpg.2017.09.005

[168] Wang J, Duan X, Li B, Jiang X. Alcohol consumption and risk of gallstone disease: A meta-analysis. European Journal of Gastroenterology & Hepatology. 2017;**29**(4):e19-e28. DOI: 10.1097/MEG.0000000000000803

[169] Cha BH, Jang M-J, Lee SH. Alcohol consumption can reduce the risk of gallstone disease: A systematic review with a dose-response meta-analysis of case-control and cohort studies. Gut Liver. 2019;**13**(1):114-131. DOI: 10.5009/gnl18278

[170] Johansson K, Sundstrom J, Marcus C, Hemmingsson E, Neovius M. Risk of symptomatic gallstones and cholecystectomy after a very-low-calorie diet or low-calorie diet in a commercial weight loss program: 1-year matched cohort study. International Journal of Obesity. 2014;**38**:279-284. DOI: 10.1038/ijo.2013.83

[171] Banim PJ, Luben RN, Bulluck H, Sharp SJ, Wareham NJ, Khaw KT, et al. The aetiology of symptomatic gallstones quantification of the effects of obesity, alcohol and serum lipids on risk. Epidemiological and biomarker data from a UK prospective cohort study (EPIC-Norfolk). European Journal of Gastroenterology & Hepatology. 2011;**23**(8):733-740. DOI: 10.1097/MEG.0b013e3283477cc9

[172] Basso L, McCollum PT, Darling MR, Tocchi A, Tanner WA. A descriptive study of pregnant women with gallstones. Relation to dietary and social habits, education, physical activity, height, and weight. European Journal of Epidemiology. 1992;**8**(5):629-633. DOI: 10.1007/BF00145375

[173] Hannuksela ML, Rantala M, Kesaniemi YA, Savolainen MJ. Ethanol-induced redistribution of cholesteryl ester transfer protein (CETP) between lipoproteins. Arteriosclerosis, Thrombosis, and Vascular Biology. 1996;**16**(2):213-221. DOI: 10.1161/01.atv.16.2.213

[174] Thornton J, Symes C, Heaton K. Moderate alcohol intake reduces bile cholesterol saturation and raises HDL cholesterol. Lancet. 1983;**2**(8354):819-822. DOI: 10.1016/s0140-6736(83)90738-9

[175] Thornton JR, Heaton KW, Macfarlane DG. A relation between high-density-lipoprotein cholesterol and bile cholesterol saturation. British Medical Journal (Clinical Research Ed.). 1981;**283**(6303):1352-1354. DOI: 10.1136/bmj.283.6303.1352

[176] Saluja AK, Bhagat L. Pathophysiology of alcohol-induced pancreatic injury. Pancreas. 2003;**27**(4):327-331. DOI: 10.1097/00006676-200311000-00010

[177] Probert C, Emmett P, Heaton K. Some determinants of whole-gut transit time: A population-based study. QJM. 1995;**88**(5):311-315

[178] Rebholz C, Krawczyk M, Lammert F. Genetics of gallstone

disease. European Journal of Clinical Investigation. 2018;**48**(7):e12935. DOI: 10.1111/eci.12935

[179] Arrese M, Cortés V, Barrera F, Nervi F. Nonalcoholic fatty liver disease, cholesterol gallstones, and cholecystectomy: New insights on a complex relationship. Current Opinion in Gastroenterology. 2018;**34**(2):90-96. DOI: 10.1097/MOG.0000000000000416

[180] Yuan S, Giovannucci EL, Larsson SC. Gallstone disease, diabetes, calcium, triglycerides, smoking and alcohol consumption and pancreatitis risk: Mendelian randomization study. NPJ Genomic Medicine. 2021;**6**(1):27. DOI: 10.1038/s41525-021-00189-6

[181] Kono S, Eguchi H, Honjo S, Todoroki I, Oda T, Shinchi K, et al. Cigarette smoking, alcohol use, and gallstone risk in Japanese men. Digestion. 2002;**65**(3):177-183. DOI: 10.1159/000064938

[182] Rhodes M, Venables C. Symptomatic gallstones-a disease of non-smokers? Digestion. 1991;**49**(4):221-226. DOI: 10.1159/000200725

[183] Tsaroucha AK, Chatzaki E, Lambropoulou M, Despoudi K, Laftsidis P, Charsou C, et al. Megalin and cubilin in the human gallbladder epithelium. Clinical and Experimental Medicine. 2008;**8**(3):165-170. DOI: 10.1007/s10238-008-0174-y

[184] Erranz B, Miquel JF, Argraves WS, Barth JL, Pimentel F, Marzolo MP. Megalin and cubilin expression in gallbladder epithelium and regulation by bile acids. Journal of Lipid Research. 2004;**45**(12):2185-2198. DOI: 10.1194/jlr.M400235-JLR200

[185] Marzolo MP, Farfán P. New insights into the roles of megalin/LRP2 and the regulation of its functional expression. Biological Research. 2011;**44**(1):89-105. DOI: 10.4067/S0716-97602011000100012

[186] Stofan M, Guo GL. Bile acids and FXR: Novel targets for liver diseases. Frontiers in Medicine (Lausanne). 2020;**7**:544. DOI: 10.3389/fmed.2020.00544

[187] Gao Q, Bi P, Mi Q, Guan Y, Jiang J, Li X, et al. Effect of nicotine on cholesterol gallstone formation in C57BL/6J mice fed on a lithogenic diet. Experimental and Therapeutic Medicine. 2023;**25**(2):84. DOI: 10.3892/etm.2023.11783

[188] Lamberts MP, Lugtenberg M, Rovers MM, et al. Persistent and de novo symptoms after cholecystectomy: A systematic review of cholecystectomy effectiveness. Surgical Endoscopy. 2013;**27**(3):709-718. DOI: 10.1007/s00464-012-2516-9

[189] Wennmacker S, Lamberts M, Gerritsen J, et al. Consistency of patient-reported outcomes after cholecystectomy and their implications on current surgical practice: A prospective multicenter cohort study. Surgical Endoscopy. 2017;**31**(1):215-224. DOI: 10.1007/s00464-016-4959-x

[190] Latenstein CSS, Wennmacker SZ, de Jong JJ, van Laarhoven CJHM, Drenth JPH, de Reuver PR. Etiologies of long-term Postcholecystectomy symptoms: A systematic review. Gastroenterology Research and Practice. 2019;**2019**:4278373. DOI: 10.1155/2019/4278373

[191] Malagelada JR, Go VL, Summerskill WH, Gamble WS. Bile acid secretion and biliary bile acid composition altered by cholecystectomy. The American Journal of Digestive Diseases. 1973;**18**:455-459. DOI: 10.1007/BF01076595

[192] Fort JM, Azpiroz F, Casellas F, Andreu J, Malagelada JR. Bowel habit after cholecystectomy: Physiological changes and clinical implications. Gastroenterology. 1996;**111**(3):617-622. DOI: 10.1053/gast.1996.v111.pm8780565

[193] Sciarretta G, Furno A, Mazzoni M, Malaguti P. Post-cholecystectomy diarrhea: Evidence of bile acid malabsorption assessed by SeHCAT test. The American Journal of Gastroenterology. 1992;**87**(12):1852-1854

[194] Yueh TP, Chen FY, Lin TE, Chuang MT. Diarrhea after laparoscopic cholecystectomy: Associated factors and predictors. Asian Journal of Surgery. 2014;**37**(4):171-177. DOI: 10.1016/j.asjsur.2014.01.008

[195] Fisher M, Spilias DC, Tong LK. Diarrhoea after laparoscopic cholecystectomy: Incidence and main determinants. ANZ Journal of Surgery. 2008;**78**(6):482-486. DOI: 10.1111/j.1445-2197.2008.04539.x

[196] Johnson AG. Gallstones and flatulent dyspepsia: Cause or coincidence? Postgraduate Medical Journal. 1971;**47**(554):767-772. DOI: 10.1136/pgmj.47.554.767

[197] Altomare DF, Rotelli MT, Palasciano N. Diet after cholecystectomy. Current Medicinal Chemistry. 2019;**26**(19):3662-3665. DOI: 10.2174/0929867324666170518100053

[198] Shin Y, Choi D, Lee KG, Choi HS, Park Y. Association between dietary intake and postlaparoscopic cholecystectomic symptoms in patients with gallbladder disease. The Korean Journal of Internal Medicine. 2018;**33**(4):829-836. DOI: 10.3904/kjim.2016.223

[199] Ribas Blasco Y, Pérez Muñante M, Gómez-Fernández L, Jovell-Fernández E, Oms Bernad LM. Low-fat diet after cholecystectomy: Should it be systematically recommended? Cirugía Española (English Edition). 2020;**98**(1):36-42. English, Spanish. DOI: 10.1016/j.ciresp.2019.05.009

[200] Marcason W. What medical nutrition therapy guideline is recommended post-cholecystectomy? Journal of the Academy of Nutrition and Dietetics. 2014;**114**(7):1136. DOI: 10.1016/j.jand.2014.05.009

[201] Burn-Murdoch RA, Fisher MA, Hunt JN. The slowing of gastric emptying by proteins in test meals. The Journal of Physiology. 1978;**274**:477-485. DOI: 10.1113/jphysiol.1978.sp012161

[202] Uchida K, Nomura Y, Kadowaki M, Takeuchi N, Yamamura Y. Effect of dietary cholesterol on cholesterol and bile acid metabolism in rats. Japanese Journal of Pharmacology. 1977;**27**(2):193-204. DOI: 10.1254/jjp.27.193

[203] Hutcheon DF, Bayless TM, Gadacz TR. Postcholecystectomy diarrhea. Journal of the American Medical Association. 1979;**241**(8):823-824

[204] Adiotomre J, Eastwood MA, Edwards CA, Brydon WG. Dietary fiber: in vitro methods that anticipate nutrition and metabolic activity in humans. The American Journal of Clinical Nutrition. 1990;**52**(1):128-134. DOI: 10.1093/ajcn/52.1.128

[205] Shim P, Choi D, Park Y. Association of blood fatty acid composition and dietary pattern with the risk of non-alcoholic fatty liver disease in patients who underwent cholecystectomy. Annals of Nutrition & Metabolism. 2017;**70**(4):303-311. DOI: 10.1159/000475605

Chapter 5

Gallbladder Stones – Pathogenesis and Treatment

Rohik Anjum, Harshavardhan Panga, Ram Prasad Subedi, Asish Das, Farhanul Huda and Navin Kumar

Abstract

Gallstone disease (GSD) refers to all the patients with symptoms due to gallstones (cholelithiasis). The presence of gallstones is a common problem seen in 10–15% of western population; with 1–4% of the population developing symptoms. The most common presentation of patients of GSD is biliary colic. There are several mechanism for cholelithiasis and all these processes are slow. Cholesterol stones are the most common variety of gallstones. Cholesterol stones cannot form if the gallbladder is completely emptied several times a day. Therefore, the total or partial extension of bile storage due to impaired gallbladder movement seems to be an important factor for cholelithiasis. Gallbladder dysmotility is an important risk factor for the development of GSD. Insufficient gallbladder motility may be associated with many risk factors for cholesterol gallstone formation, such as pregnant women, obese patients, and their rapid weight loss, diabetes mellitus, and patients receiving total parenteral nutrition. Transabdominal ultrasound is the mainstay in the evaluation of patients with GSD. The presence of gallbladder dysfunction can be studied using cholecystokinin (CCK)-stimulated cholescintigraphy to evaluate for gallbladder ejection fraction (GBEF); with values <40% after 30 mins of CCK infusion considered diagnostic. The definitive treatment of GSD is cholecystectomy.

Keywords: gallstone disease, cholelithiasis, pathogenesis of gallstones, gallbladder dysmotility, cholecystectomy

1. Introduction

Gallstone disease (GSD) is one of the most common diseases affecting 10–15% of adult population. Out of this, 80% of the individuals are asymptomatic and the disease is detected incidentally while performing abdominal ultrasound for any other pathology or during screening. The asymptomatic patients may eventually experience symptoms ~2–3% per year, reaching up to 10% by 5 years. The complicated GSD affects 1–2% of patients with GSD [1]. The complications of GSD include cholecystitis, pancreatitis and gallbladder cancer. The incidence of GSD is more in female gender and increases with age. The formation of gallstones are multifactorial. There are some local factors in the gallbladder, which include dysmotility of the gallbladder, inflammation of gallbladder wall and mucin accumulation in the gallbladder. Other local factor is in the bile, which consists of supersaturation of cholesterol. Bile contains mixed micelles which are composed of cholesterol, phospholipid and bile salts. The bile is thermodynamically stable under the action of mixed micelles and cholesterol does not precipitate. There is variation in the relative concentration of cholesterol in bile. When the cholesterol is supersaturated in the bile then precipitation of cholesterol happens, which forms the cholesterol gall stones. Cholesterol stones are the most common variety of gallstones. There are some systemic factors which include expression and activity of nuclear receptors, hormonal factors (insulin resistance), altered cholesterol metabolism, altered intestinal motility and gut microbiota [2]. Surgery is the mainstay in the treatment of symptomatic GSD or gallstones with complications.

2. Risk factors and pathogenesis

The pathogenesis of gallstones are multifactorial including a variety of genetic and environmental factors. The risk factors for gallstones are modifiable and non-modifiable. The age, sex, race, and genetic factors are nonmodifiable whereas metabolic syndrome, intestinal microflora disorders, impaired gallbladder motility, and immune disorders are important modifiable factors. Pathogenesis of gallstones include local factors in the gallbladder and bile, and systemic factors like elevated proinflammatory proteins (interleukin-6,10,12,13) [2–4]. The local factors in the gall bladder include gallbladder dysmotility, hypersecretion and accumulation of mucin gel in the gall bladder lumen. The local factors in the bile consists of rapid phase transition of cholesterol from supersaturated hepatic bile and local immune mediated inflammation in the gallbladder [2].

2.1 Age and sex

The gallstones are more common in older individuals and in female gender. Increased incidence in female is because of influence of estrogen on cholesterol metabolism.

2.2 Family history

Family history of gallstones increases the risk of development of GSD. A Swedish study done on twins in 43,141 patients showed that 25% of risk of GSD is determined by the underlying genetic predisposition [5]. These studies confirmed specific gene polymorphism in the formation of gallstones but the environmental factors including diet and physical activity have also the crucial role [6–11].

2.3 Pregnancy

Pregnancy is a risk factor for the development of cholesterol stones. This is due to change in the bile composition and delayed gallbladder emptying, which promotes the formation of gallstones.

2.4 Metabolic causes

Elevated non-HDL cholesterol (dyslipedemia) is associated with increased risk of gallstones. Diabetes mellitus is also associated with an increased risk of cholesterol gallstones. Insulin resistance appears to be an important cause for GSD [12].

2.5 Obesity

Obesity has been established as a risk factor for the development of cholesterol gallstones. This is due to enhanced cholesterol synthesis and secretion. The risk of development of gallstones seems to be higher in females, especially in those with morbid obesity [13].

2.6 Rapid weight loss

Higher rates of gallstones have been reported to be associated with rapid weight loss; especially those on very low calories (diet with <800 kcal/day) or after gastric bypass. The exact mechanism by which weight loss cause gallstones are not known, however, the levels of biliary mucin and biliary calcium levels have been noted to be much higher compared to the general population; these factors may promote cholesterol nucleation and gallstone formation [14].

2.7 Drugs associated with formation of gallstones

Some drugs are associated with the development of gallstones like fibrates, somatostatin analogues, hormone replacement and OCPs.

2.8 Conditions causing gallbladder stasis

Prolonged fasting and treatment with parenteral nutrition are associated with increased gallbladder stasis. The cause of biliary stasis is attributed to the lack of enteral stimulation of gallbladder and lack of enterohepatic circulation of bile acids in patients with ileal resection. Interruption of the enterohepatic circulation of bile acids results in the reduction of hepatic bile acids and resulting in increased lithogenicity of hepatic bile, which tends to become supersaturated with cholesterol. Normal gallbladder absorbs the water from bile making it concentrated. Due to gallbladder stasis the bile becomes overly saturated with cholesterol, causing gallstone formation.

2.9 Gallbladder dysmotility

This entity is considered as a risk factor for the development of GSD. The cause of gallstone in dysmotility may be attributed to gallbladder stasis. Gallbladder dysmotility in some cases may be attributed to decreased sensitivity of gallbladder to cholecystokinin (CCK) [15]. Defective intrinsic innervation causes marked reduction in the neurons and interstitial cells of cajal like cells (ICLCs) in the gallbladder. They have a role in the motility of the gallbladder. It has been observed that ICLCs density is markedly reduced in the gallbladder with stones. The reduced density of ICLCs decreases the gallbladder motility [16].

2.10 Immune disorders

Cholesterol secretion is increased by inflammatory mediators. These mediators promote lipid secretion and metabolism in liver. It causes cholesterol supersaturation in the bile. Bile contains low concentration of various immunoglobulins including IgA, IgG and IgM. The IgM is most effective in the gallstone formation in supersaturated bile [17].

2.11 Intestinal microflora disorder

Studies showed that the caecum of the patient with gall stones have increased number of gram positive anaerobes with increased 7α-dehydroxylation activity. These causes increased concentration of deoxycholate (secondary bile acid) which is more hydrophobic and lithogenic [18].

3. Types of gallstones

The gallstones are usually composed of a mixture of cholesterol, calcium salts of bilirubinate or palmitate, proteins, and mucin. The gallstones are mainly classified into 3 groups- cholesterol stones, black pigment stones and brown pigment stones. Cholesterol stones are the most common variety of stones usually seen in patients with genetic or environmental predispositions. These stones occur due to the supersaturation of bile with cholesterol and consist of calcium salts of bilirubinate and palmitate. Black pigment stones are usually found in patients with hemolysis and consist primarily of calcium bilirubinate. The brown pigment stones are found in association with bacterial or parasitic infection of the biliary system. They may also be found in the bile ducts due to biliary system manipulation. Regarding the prevalence of the type of gallstones, the most common variety is the cholesterol stones accounting for ~75% of gallstones, black stones accounting for 20% and brown stones accounting for 5% [19].

4. Pathophysiology of gallstone formation

The mechanism of gallstone formation amongst the various types of gallstones are mentioned below.

4.1 Cholesterol gallstone formation

The main route of cholesterol excretion from the body is via biliary secretion. Cholesterol is a hydrophobic molecule, which is relatively insoluble in bile. Bile salts and phospholipids are incorporated in micelles with cholesterol to increase their solubility. The excess cholesterol is usually kept in vesicles (not in micelle). These vesicles usually contain cholesterol with phospholipids. The vesicle cholesterol nucleation occurs when they get supersaturated with cholesterol. Vesicles are said to be super saturated when the vesicle cholesterol/phospholipid ratio is >1 [20]. The supersaturated vesicles may get aggregated from unilamellar to multilamellar vesicles and later the process of cholesterol crystal nucleation occurs. The bile is concentrated 3–4 folds in the gallbladder due to water absorption and progressively increasing cholesterol in the micelle due to the preferential solubilization of bile salts with phospholipids leaving supersaturated bile cause cholesterol nucleation and this explains why the gallstones are usually seen in gallbladder than anywhere else in the biliary tree. There are some factors that can further promote gallstone formation like IgM, IgG, haptoglobins, alpha-1 acid glycoprotein, alpha-1 antichymotrysin and mucin, based on various invitro and in vivo studies [21]. Gallbladder dysmotility is another important factor for the development of cholesterol nucleation, since it causes stagnation of bile leading to crystal aggregation.

4.2 Black pigment stone formation

The black pigment stones are formed in cases of haemolytic anemia. They are primarily composed of calcium bilirubinate and tend to occur due to high levels of bilirubin (10-fold) which are excreted in bile due to haemolysis [22].

4.3 Brown pigment stone formation

The brown pigment stones are primarily seen in bacterial infection of the bile ducts by organisms such as E. Coli, Bacteroides, Clostridium, Clonorchis sinensis, and Ascaris lumbricoides. These organisms produce the enzyme, Beta glucuronidase, phospholipase A, and bile acid hydrolase which lead to increased amounts of unconjugated bilirubin which combine with calcium resulting in stone formation. The parasites may stimulate stones formation by the presence of calcified eggs, which may serve as a nidus and enhance the precipitation of calcium bilirubinate [23].

5. Clinical features

Most individuals with the presence of gallstones are asymptomatic, usually diagnosed on screening imaging. The most common presenting symptoms of patients of GSD is abdominal pain, termed as biliary colic (**Table 1**). It typically starts as a dull discomfort in the right upper abdomen, severe in intensity with radiation to the back. It is usually associated with diaphoresis, nausea, and vomiting. The term biliary colic is considered as a misnomer since the pain is usually constant and not colicky. The pain in biliary colic usually lasts 30 minutes, plateauing in an hour and starts to subside. The episode of pain in biliary colic usually lasts <6 hours [24]. The pain is classically triggered by a fatty meal, which causes gallbladder contraction with cystic duct blocked by stones, leading to increase pressure inside the gallbladder. However, this association is not universal [25]. The pain subsides when the gallbladder relaxes, leading to the stones blocking the cystic duct to fall back into the gallbladder. Some individuals can also present with atypical symptoms such as bloating, belching, nausea, vomiting or abdominal distention. Few patients of GSD may also present with complications related to gallstones like cholecystitis, choledocholithiasis, cholangitis, gallstone induced pancreatitis, Mirizzi syndrome or gallstone ileus. The important definitions regarding the presentation of gallstones diseases are mentioned in **Table 2**.

• Pain in the epigastrium or right upper quadrant
• Increase in severity over 30 minutes
• Pain plateaus within an hour
• Duration lasts <6 hours
• Severe enough to disrupt routine activities or lead to hospital visits
• Interval of symptoms can be variable.
• Association with food intake (especially fatty meals)

Table 1.
Features of classical biliary pain in GSD.

• Cholelithiasis/cholecystolithiasis	• Refers to the presence of stones in the gallbladder
• GSD	• Refers to gallstones causing symptoms
• Uncomplicated GSD	• Refers to GSD without gallstone-related complications
• Complicated GSD	• Refers to the GSD with gallstone-related complications like acute cholecystitis, acute cholangitis, gallstone induced pancreatitis, Mirizzi syndrome and gallstone ileus.

Table 2.
Definitions related to gallstones used in clinical practice.

6. Investigations

The main investigation for the diagnosis of GSD is transabdominal ultrasonography. Endoscopic ultrasonography is an alternative investigation done for cases where the sensitivity of transabdominal ultrasound in low (gallstones <3 mm). Computed tomography, oral cholecystography and cholescintigraphy (HIDA scan) are tests which are done in some special circumstance, like those planned for dissolution therapy (**Table 3**).

• Imaging modality	• Salient features
• USG abdomen	• Preliminary investigation of choice • Smaller stones (<3 mm) may be missed
• Computed tomography	• Non-contrast CT can assess the stone composition. • Floating stones (buoyancy) indicates high cholesterol concentration [26]. • Low density (black holes) suggests cholesterol stones. • Stones with density < 75 HU are susceptible to dissolution; whereas stones >100 HU dissolve poorly [27]. • Highly calcified stones are unlikely to dissolve. • If gallstones are not visualized on CT, it means the stones are isodense to bile. CT density of bile in these cases helps predict the outcome.
• Oral cholecystography	• Can help in the assessment of number, size, buoyance, cystic duct patency and gallbladder concentration ability. • Oral contrast agents (eg: iopanoic acid) are administered the night before. • Visualization of the gallbladder suggests adequate intestinal absorption, secretion into bile by the liver and concentration in the gallbladder. • Can indirectly measure motor function by the reduction in the size of the gallbladder on serial radiographs after a fatty meal. • Gallstone buoyancy can be seen as suggestive of cholesterol stones
• Cholescintigraphy (HIDA scan)	• Can be used to identify cystic duct patency. • Mucosal function cannot be assessed as the concentration of the tracer in the gallbladder is not needed for visualization, unlike oral cholecystography.

Table 3.
Summary of investigations to be done before gallstone dissolution therapy.

DOI: http://dx.doi.org/10.5772/intechopen.1002259

6.1 Transabdominal ultrasound

Transabdominal ultrasound is the most common investigation performed for the diagnosis of GSD. It is readily available, non-invasive, and does not subject the patient to the harmful effects of ionizing radiation. Overnight fasting or fasting for 8 hours before the ultrasound evaluation of the gallbladder is recommended for distension of the gallbladder with bile. This helps in better visualization of gallstones. The stones are visible as echogenic contents within the lumen of the gallbladder with posterior acoustic shadowing (**Figure 1**). These tend to be usually mobile and deposit according to gravity. Biliary sludge is usually echogenic, but does not cast posterior acoustic shadows. Gallbladder polyps on the other hand have a similar appearance as gallstones but do not cast posterior acoustic shadow. The sensitivity of detecting gallstones by USG is 76–99% and specificity is 99% [28]. However, it has been noted that the sensitivity of gallstones reduces to 50–60% for gallstones <3 mm in size [29].

6.2 Endoscopic ultrasound

Endoscopic ultrasound (EUS) is useful in select few cases of GSD. It is a useful investigation to detect small gallstones (<3 mm) which may be missed on transabdominal ultrasound and in obese patients with difficult visualization of gallstones. EUS also has the added benefit of visualization of the gastric and duodenal mucosa which helps in the diagnosis of peptic ulcer disease, which may mimic the symptoms of GSD. The sensitivity of EUS for the detection of GSD is 96% and the specificity is 86% [30].

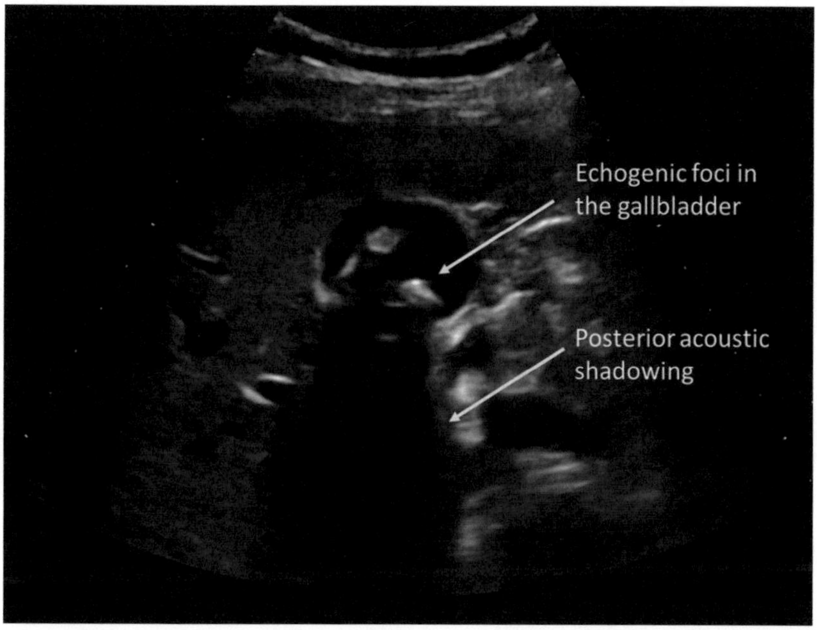

Figure 1.
Shows the presence of gallstones in the gallbladder. Echogenic foci in the gallbladder with posterior acoustic shadowing.

7. Prevention of gallstone disease

7.1 Dietary and lifestyle modification

The aim is to maintain the ideal body weight and maintain healthy lifestyle. The following are recommended:

- Eating three well balanced diet containing adequate fiber and low in saturated fats. Regular meal timing prevents gallbladder stasis of bile and ensures adequate emptying.
- Gradual weight reduction of <1.5 kg/month is recommended for obese individuals. Diet containing <800 kcal/day is not recommended.
- Regular exercise will help to maintain the body weight.
- Enteral feeds are always recommended over parenteral. Patients who are on parenteral nutrition should be periodically assessed for the resumption of enteral nutrition.
- Diets rich in poly and monounsaturated fats inhibits cholesterol gallstone formation and thus reduce the risk of the development of gallstones [31].
- Coffee consumption has been associated with decreased risk of developing gallstones. The exact mechanism is not known, probably attributed its effect on cholesterol gallstone formation [32].

7.2 Ursodeoxycholic acid supplementation

Ursodeoxycholic acid (UDCA) is recommended for the prevention of gallstones due to rapid weight loss in patients undergoing bariatric procedures. A dose of 600 mg/day is usually given in two divided doses. Studies suggest a significant reduction in the rate of gallstone formation in such patients from ~28% in the placebo group to 3% in patients on 600 mg/day of the drug [33]. UDCA acts by reducing the intestinal absorption of cholesterol and improving gallbladder emptying. It is also used for gallstone dissolution because of its ability to dissolve the cholesterol in gallstones [34].

7.3 Vitamin C supplementation

Vitamin C may have a protective effect on gallstones. The exact mechanism of action is not known but it is postulated to be due to its effects on the conversion of cholesterol to bile acid [35].

8. Management of gallstone disease

All patients with symptomatic gallstones are advised for laparoscopic cholecystectomy, this includes both uncomplicated and complicated GSD. The timing of surgery is maybe decided based on individual patient and surgeon preferences. The debate on the management of patients with asymptomatic gallstones rages on. The current

1. Gallbladder adenomas
2. Large gallstones (>3 mm)
3. Porcelain gallbladder
4. Longer duration (>40 years)
5. Regions with higher incidence like Chile, Bolivia, South Korea, China and North India [36]

Table 4.
Gallstones with increased risk of gallbladder cancer.

consensus is to perform cholecystectomy for asymptomatic patients who are at increased risk of gallbladder cancer (**Table 4**) [37]. The patients who are unwilling for surgery or those not fit for surgery may be considered for non-surgical management. The details of this are mentioned in the subsequent section.

8.1 Non-surgical management

Non-surgical management of GSD is mainly done in asymptomatic patients whereas cholecystectomy is the treatment of choice in symptomatic gallstones. Non-surgical management of gallstones is theoretically safer owing to the avoidance of general anesthesia and surgical risk; however, these need patients to follow up at regular intervals, high rates of treatment failure and recurrences and the dissolution therapy for gallstones mainly works for cholesterol stones. The candidates for successful gallstone dissolution therapy are mentioned in **Table 5**. Prospective multicentre trials done on gallstone dissolution in South Korea shows a response rate of close to 50% in 6 months with the administration of UDCA [38]. Pre-treatment imaging is recommended before the initiation of dissolution therapy. The main aim of the imaging is to evaluate the composition of gallstones, number and size of the stones, patency of cystic duct and the concentrating capacity of the gallbladder. Radioluscency is an important factor for the decision of dissoluation therapy. CT scan is important before the start of dissolution therapy, since <50% of gallstones which were radioluscent on abdominal radiograph, turn out to be hyperdense on CT; thereby not fit for gallstone dissolution therapy. The summary of pre-treatment imaging in mentioned in **Table 3**.

8.1.1 Gallstone dissolution therapy

After the proper selection of patients for dissolution therapy (**Table 5**), treatment with UDCA is initiated. It is given at a dose of 10 mg/kg daily in 2 divided

• Small gallstones (<1 cm)
• Cholesterol stones
• Radiolucent on plane abdominal X-ray
• Uncomplicated GSD
• Patent cystic duct
• Normal functioning gallbladder

Table 5.
Gallstone dissolution therapy.

doses. It acts by dissolving the cholesterol from both the surface and the center of the gallstone. It also inhibits the intestinal absorption of cholesterol and improves the gallbladder emptying functions [34]. The calcium in the stones disintegrates subsequently and is expelled by the contraction of the gallbladder. The cystic duct must be patent for the drug to enter the gallbladder. Normal gallbladder mucosa must be functional to absorb the water and to concentrate the drug in the gallbladder; needed for its ability to dissolve the gallstone. Adequate contraction of the gallbladder is needed for the dissolve cholesterol and the stone debris to be expelled from the gallbladder. The dosage of UDCA is given in divided doses since it helps maintain the drug biliary concentration levels and help in increased stone dissolution. A study done comparing UDCA and a combination of UDCA with Cheno-deoxycholic acid (CDCA) in Korea shows comparable results for gallstone dissolution [39]. CDCA also has more incidence with diarrhea, hypercholesterolemia and an increase in liver transaminase levels [40]. Hence, UDCA is the recommended drug of choice for gallstone dissolution therapy. The follow-up of patients on dissolution therapy is kept every 6 months to 1 year to assess for its response. It must be remembered that most gallstones dissolve from the inside out, hence the size of follow-up may not decrease drastically before the external shell of the gallstone disintegrates. The drug is also continued for 6 months after the complete dissolution of gallstones. The standard rate of gallstone dissolution is 1 mm/month [41]. Multiple small stones dissolve faster than a single large stone due to greater surface area. In a typical patient planned for dissolution therapy (noncalcified small cholesterol stones with functioning gallbladder), the dissolution rates are >90% [42]. However, only 10% of individuals with gallstones are fit for dissolution therapy. Multicentric studies by the British-Italian Gallstone study group found a mean dissolution of 47% in 6 months and at 12 months. Complete dissolution of gallstones was found in around 30% of patients by 1 year [40].

8.2 Surgical treatment: cholecystectomy

8.2.1 Surgical anatomy of gallbladder

The gallbladder is located below segment IVb and V of liver. It is a pear-shaped organ which accommodates ~30 cc of bile but can collect upto ~50 cc of bile. The gallbladder normally has three parts—fundus, body, and the neck (infundibulum). The surface landmark of the gallbladder is at the 9th costal cartilage; at the junction of lateral border of rectus abdominis and the costal margin. The neck of the gallbladder opens into the cystic duct, which in turn open into the bile duct. A pathological part of gallbladder is known as the hartmann's pouch which is an outpouching of the neck of the gallbladder due to gallstones. The cystic duct is about 2–4 cm long and 1–3 mm wide; it is <2 cm in length in 20% of individuals [43]. The mucosa of cystic duct is spirally folded to form the valves of heister. These valves are thought to provide support to the wall of cystic duct and prevent its collapse [44]. Sphincter of the cystic duct is called the sphincter of lutkens; which help to regulate the flow of bile from the gallbladder. The gallbladder is supplied by the cystic artery, branch of right hepatic artery. Moynihan's hump is seen in ~15% of individuals, where the right hepatic artery forms a loop and is found close to the gallbladder, thereby mistaking it for cystic artery (**Figure 2**) [45]. Various variations in biliary and vascular anatomy have been described.

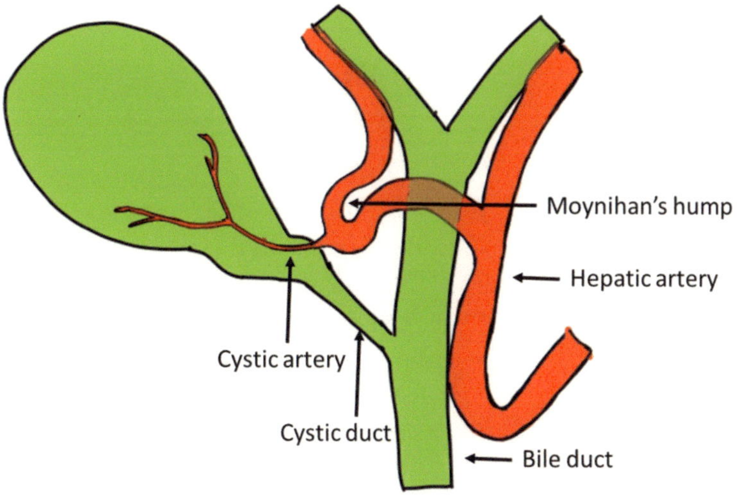

Figure 2.
Shows the presence of Moynihan's hump with short cystic artery. (The right hepatic artery can be easily mistaken for the cystic artery and divided.)

8.2.2 Laparoscopic cholecystectomy

Laparoscopic cholecystectomy is considered as the gold standard surgery for cholelithiasis. Indications for cholecystectomy have been illustrated in **Table 6**. the procedure is done under general anesthesia. Nasogastric tube decompression is done, and bladder emptying is ensured.

The standard port positions in laparoscopic cholecystectomy are shown in **Figure 3**. The umbilical port is placed either by the veress needle technique or the open technique. The other three ports are placed under direct vision after the creation of the pneumoperitoneum. The position of the patient is then turned to reverse Trendelenburg position with the right side up.

- In North America, the surgeon stands at the patient's left and the assistant to the right of the patient. The camera person stands to the left of the operating surgeon.

- In Europe, the patient is in a supine position with abducted legs. The surgeons stand between the legs of the patient, the camera person stands to the left and the assistant stands to the right of the patient.

• Symptomatic cholelithiasis
• Asymptomatic cholelithiasis in patients with increased risk of complications/malignancy.
• Acalculous cholecystitis
• Gallbladder polyp >10 mm
• Porcelain gallbladder

Table 6.
Indications of cholecystectomy.

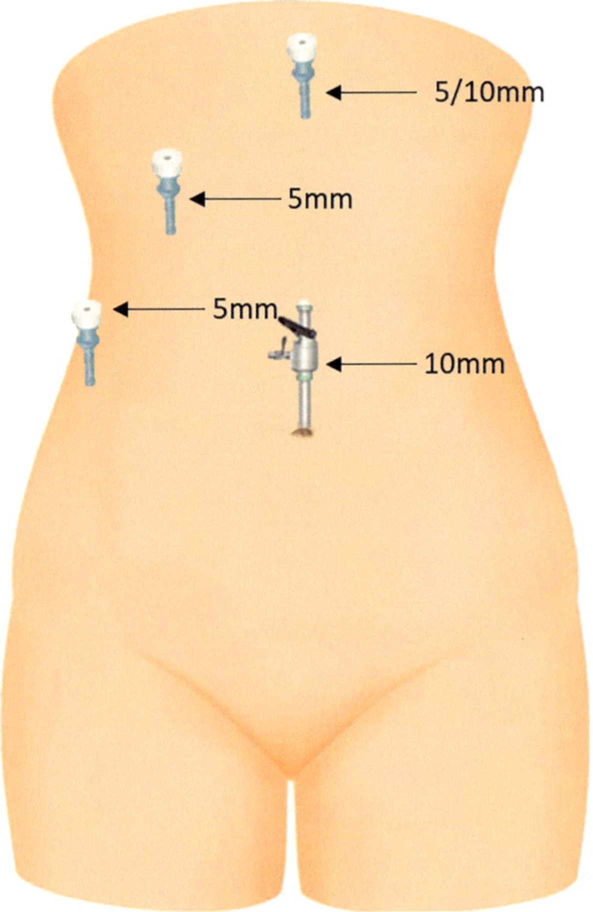

Figure 3.
Shows the port placement in laparoscopic cholecystectomy.

Dissection steps:

1. Gallbladder exposure—The gallbladder is dissected from adhesions to the omentum, duodenum, and colon. The assistant retracts the gallbladder superior and laterally using a grasper. If the gallbladder is distended and difficult to aspiration; a wide bore needle is inserted into the gallbladder and the bile is aspirated.

2. Dissection of hepatocystic triangle—The hepatocystic triangle is bounded by the cytstic duct, inferior edge of liver and the common hepatic duct. All the fibrofatty tissue is cleared from the triangle. If a large stone is blocking the neck of gallbladder, it may be pushed into the gallbladder for easier dissection. The operating surgeon must hold the infundibulum and retract it infero-laterally. The posterior dissection will need the surgeon to retract the infundibulum supero-medially. The rouvier's sulcus is a fissure between the right lobe and the caudate process of liver. This corresponds to the level of porta where the right pedicle enters the liver. The recommendation is to stay superior the rouvier sulcus for safety [46]. R4U line has been described by Gupta and Jain [47], connecting the

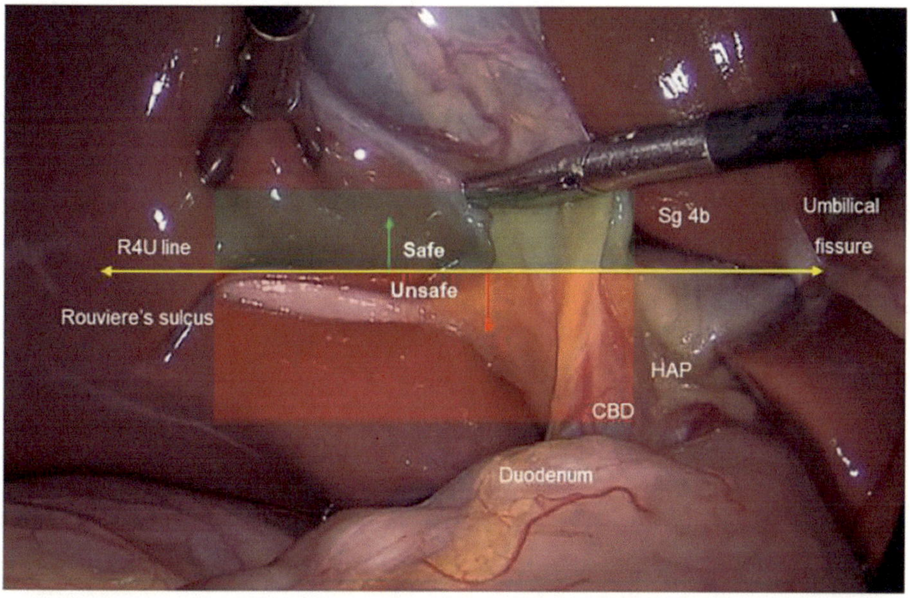

Figure 4.
Show the R4U line connecting the rouviere's sulcus to base of segment IV until the umbilical fissure. The dissection is recommended to be done above this plane.

rouvier sulcus, base of segment IV up to the umbilical fissure. The dissection is recommended to be done above this line for safety (**Figure 4**).

3. Achieving the critical view of safety—The critical view of safety by proposed by Strasberg in 1995 to promote the accurate recognition of structures during laparoscopic cholecystectomy and to prevent the occurrence of bile duct injury [48]. It is also recognized as part of Society of American Gastrointestinal and Endoscopic Surgeons (SAGES) and incorporated in the "Safe cholecystectomy program". The details of critical view of safety have been shown in **Table 7**, (**Figure 5**). The operating surgeon should be aware of the common variations in the bilio-vascular anatomy.

4. Division of the cystic artery and duct—The cystic artery and the cystic duct are fully dissected. The cystic artery is first clipped and divided (two clips proximally and one clip distally towards the gallbladder). The cystic artery gives of an anterior and posterior branch, usually close to the gallbladder; however, in some cases the branching takes place proximally, in such cases the anterior branch may

• There are three components to the critical view of safety: 1. Hepatocystic triangle is cleared of fibrofatty tissue (to note: the CBD and the CHD do not have to be exposed). 2. Lower third of gallbladder is separated from the cystic plate. 3. Two and only two structures should be seen entering the gallbladder.

Table 7.
Critical view of safety.

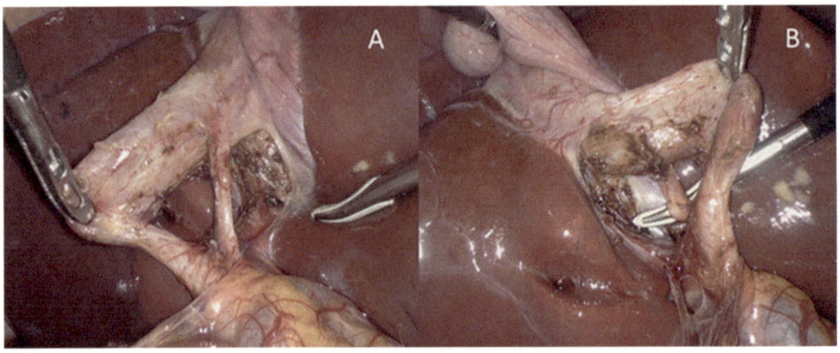

Figure 5.
Duplet view of critical view of safety: (a) anterior; (b) posterior.

be divided instead of posteriorly. Hence the posterior branch must be looked, if not appreciated can result in troublesome bleeds during cholecystectomy. The cystic duct is then milked retrograde to push any stones if present in the cystic duct into the gallbladder. The cystic duct is clipped and divided. Intraoperative cholangiography can be done at this step if any doubt in the biliary anatomy exists. Some of the tips shown in **Table 8** that can be followed in difficult situations during laparoscopic cholecystectomy.

5. Dissection of the gallbladder from liver bed- the gallbladder is then dissected away from the liver bed using hook or spatula cautery. If the dissection is done in the correct plane, there is usually minimal bleeding. Prior to detachment of gallbladder from the liver bed, the liver is inspected for any bleeding or bile leak. The right upper quadrant is irrigated and suctioned. The gallbladder is then fully detached from the liver surface.

6. Gallbladder extraction: the gallbladder is extracted either from the 10 mm epigastric port or the 10 mm umbilical port. An extraction bag may be used if the gallbladder is inflamed, friable or perforated. After the extraction, the right upper quadrant maybe further irrigated and suctioned. Hemostasis and no bile leak is ensured. The trocars are removed under direct vision and the 10 mm trocar sites are closed using appropriate sutures. The skin is approximated using sutures or staplers. The access sites local anesthesia may be used.

• Tips to follow in difficult situations
• Thorough knowledge of the anatomy and variation must be known.
• A good vision by a good laparoscope
• Obtain critical view of safety whenever possible.
• Recognize the safe and unsafe areas.
• Make liberal use of cholangiography whenever required.
• Intraoperative momentary pause before clipping or dividing.
• Get help from colleague or seniors in difficult situations.

Table 8.
Tips to followed during laparoscopic cholecystectomy.

8.2.3 SILS cholecystectomy

Single incision laparoscopic surgery (SILS) cholecystectomy makes use of a single incision for the surgery. Laparoscope with specially made instruments are used for this procedure. This was first reported by Navarra et al. [49] in 1997 using transabdominal sutures to retract the gallbladder. For retraction traction sutures may be used according to the surgeon discretion. The steps of cholecystectomy are like the standard 4 port cholecystectomy and the specimen is extracted using a specimen retraction bag via the umbilical port. The facial defect must be carefully closed to prevent incisional hernia in future [50]. A preliminary study done in 2012 comparing the SILS to traditional laparoscopic cholecystectomy shows slightly longer operative time (~65 minutes) compared to 4 port laparoscopic cholecystectomy which may be attributable to the learning curve of the procedure. Metanalysis done in 2022 comparing SILS to the standard laparoscopic cholecystectomy shows less immediate postoperative pain in the group; but similar pain on days 1 and 2 of the procedure, longer operative time, and more complications than in conventional 4 port laparoscopic cholecystectomy. Complications including bile leak, intra-abdominal collection, and surgical site wound infection were found to be higher in the SILS group. Conversion from laparoscopy to open surgery was similar in both groups [51]. Hence, this is an alternative technique of laparoscopic cholecystectomy and further studies are warranted for the evolution of the technique.

8.2.4 NOTES cholecystectomy

Natural orifice transluminal endoscopic surgery (NOTES) cholecystectomy, via transvaginal approach, has gained some popularity in recent years. Ricardo Zorron from Brazil in 2007 published the first report on transvaginal hybrid notes [52]. The procedure is done by placing the laparoscope (10 mm) via the posterior vagina and 5 mm umbilical port. The access may be done through the stomach, urinary bladder, or colon. The critical view of safety may be slightly different compared to a standard 4-port laparoscopic cholecystectomy owing to a different viewing angle. However, the cystic artery and the duct are dissected and clipped like the laparoscopic technique. It must be noted some challenges might be encountered during specimen extraction from the vagina using the specimen retrieval bag. Meta-analysis comparing the NOTES cholecystectomy with the laparoscopic cholecystectomy shows no significant difference regarding the safety of the procedure or wound complications. It was noted that the operating time for NOTES cholecystectomy was significantly longer than laparoscopic cholecystectomy by around 34 minutes; however, the postoperative pain was less in the NOTES cholecystectomy group [53]. Hence, this is an alternative technique of cholecystectomy, however, needs good procedural training, specially designed surgical instruments, and further studies to validate for general use.

8.2.5 Robotic surgery (robotic assisted cholecystectomy)

Robotic surgery has many advantages including the 3D view, enhanced instrument articulation, intraoperative fluorescence imaging and precise movements. Docking of the robot is done, and the steps of surgery are like the laparoscopic surgery. Studies done comparing laparoscopy with robotic surgery show longer operative time for robotic surgery with comparable conversion and complication rates. There was also no significant difference in the length of hospital stay, surgical site infection or readmissions. However, it has to be mentioned that the hospital costs of robotic surgery are significantly higher than that of laparoscopic surgery [54].

9. Conclusion

GSD is one of the most common diseases affecting 10-15% of adult population. Eighty percent of these individuals are asymptomatic. Biliary colic is the most common presentation. Pathogenesis of the gallstones are multifactorial which include non-modifiable and modifiable factors. Cholesterol stones are the most common variety of gallstones. Cholesterol gallstones cannot form if the gallbladder is completely emptied several times a day. Therefore, gallbladder dysmotility seems to be an important factor for cholelithiasis. Gallbladder dysmotility may be attributed to decreased sensitivity of the gallbladder to CCK. It has been observed that ICLCs density is markedly reduced in the gallbladder with stones. The reduced density of ICLCs decreases the gallbladder motility. Transabdominal ultrasound is the mainstay in the evaluation of patients with GSD. The presence of gallbladder dysfunction can be studied using CCK-stimulated cholescintigraphy to evaluate for gallbladder ejection fraction (GBEF); with values <40% after 30 mins of CCK infusion considered diagnostic. The definitive treatment of GSD is cholecystectomy and laparoscopic cholecystectomy is considered as gold standard.

Conflict of interest

The authors declare no conflict of interest.

Author details

Rohik Anjum, Harshavardhan Panga, Ram Prasad Subedi, Asish Das, Farhanul Huda and Navin Kumar*
Department of Surgery, All India Institute of Medical Sciences, Rishikesh, India

*Address all correspondence to: navin.surg@aiimsrishikesh.edu.in

References

[1] Stinton LM, Shaffer EA. Epidemiology of gallbladder disease: cholelithiasis and cancer. Gut Liver. 2012;**6**(2):172-187

[2] Di Ciaula A, Portincasa P. Recent advances in understanding and managing cholesterol gallstones. F1000Research 2018;7(F1000 Faculty Rev):1529

[3] Di Ciaula A, Wang DQH, Portincasa P. An update on the pathogenesis of cholesterol gallstone disease. Current Opinion in Gastroenterology. 2018;**34**(2):71-80

[4] Liu Z, Kemp TJ, Gao YT, et al. Association of circulating inflammation proteins and gallstone disease. Journal of Gastroenterology and Hepatology. 2018;**33**(11):1920-1924

[5] Katsika D, Grjibovski A, Einarsson C, Lammert F, Lichtenstein P, Marschall HU. Genetic and environmental influences on symptomatic gallstone disease: a Swedish study of 43,141 twin pairs. Hepatology. 2005;**41**(5):1138-1143

[6] Martinez-Lopez E, Curiel-Lopez F, Hernandez-Nazara A, et al. Influence of ApoE and FABP2 polymorphisms and environmental factors in the susceptibility to gallstone disease. Annals of Hepatology. 2015;**14**(4):515-523

[7] Di Ciaula A, Garruti G, Frühbeck G, et al. The role of diet in the pathogenesis of cholesterol gallstones. Current Medicinal Chemistry. 2019;**26**(19):3620-3638

[8] Di Ciaula A, Portincasa P. Diet and contaminants: driving the rise to obesity epidemics? Current Medicinal Chemistry. 2019;**26**(19):3471-3482

[9] Stokes CS, Krawczyk M, Lammert F. Gallstones: environment, lifestyle and genes. Digestive Diseases. 2011;**29**(2):191-201

[10] Unisa S, Jagannath P, Dhir V, et al. Population-based study to estimate prevalence and determine risk factors of gallbladder diseases in the rural gangetic basin of North India. HPB: The Official Journal of the International Hepato Pancreato Biliary Association. 2011;**13**(2):117-125

[11] Parviainen A, Suárez-Grau JM, Pérez-López R, et al. Combined microstructural and mineralogical phase characterization of gallstones in a patient-based study in SW Spain - implications for environmental contamination in their formation. Science of the Total Environment. 2016;**573**:433-443

[12] Biddinger SB, Haas JT, Yu BB, Bezy O, Jing E, Zhang W, et al. Hepatic insulin resistance directly promotes formation of cholesterol gallstones. Nature Medicine. 2008;**14**(7):778-782

[13] Stampfer MJ, Maclure KM, Colditz GA, Manson JE, Willett WC. Risk of symptomatic gallstones in women with severe obesity. The American Journal of Clinical Nutrition. 1992;**55**(3):652-658

[14] Shiffman ML, Kaplan GD, Brinkman-Kaplan V, Vickers FF. Prophylaxis against gallstone formation with ursodeoxycholic acid in patients participating in a very-low-calorie diet program. Annals of Internal Medicine. 1995;**122**(12):899-905

[15] Jonkers IJ, Smelt AH, Ledeboer M, Hollum ME, Biemond I, Kuipers F, et al. Gall bladder dysmotility: a risk factor for gall stone formation in hypertriglyceridaemia and reversal

on triglyceride lowering therapy by bezafibrate and fish oil. Gut. 2003;**52**(1):109-115

[16] Franks I. Loss of interstitial Cajal-like cells in the gallbladder might contribute to gallstone formation. Nature Reviews. Gastroenterology & Hepatology. 2012;**9**:689

[17] Reynoso-Paz S, Coppel RL, Mackay IR, Bass NM, Ansari AA, Gershwin ME. The immunobiology of bile and biliary epithelium. Hepatology. 1999;**30**:351-357

[18] Thomas LA, Veysey MJ, Murphy GM, et al. Octreotide induced prolongation of colonic transit increases faecal anaerobic bacteria, bile acid metabolizing enzymes, and serum deoxycholic acid in patients with acromegaly. Gut. 2005;**54**(5):630-635

[19] Attili AF, Capocaccia R, Carulli N, Festi D, Roda E, Barbara L, et al. Factors associated with gallstone disease in the MICOL experience. Multicenter Italian Study on Epidemiology of Cholelithiasis. Hepatology. 1997;**26**(4):809-818

[20] Somjen GJ, Gilat T. Contribution of vesicular and micellar carriers to cholesterol transport in human bile. Journal of Lipid Research. 1985;**26**:699-704

[21] Wang DQ, Cohen DE, Carey MC. Biliary lipids and cholesterol gallstone disease. Journal of Lipid Research. 2009;**50**(Suppl):S406-S411

[22] Rambaud E, Ranque B, Pouchot J, Arlet JB. Complications lithiasiques chez les patients drépanocytaires [Gallstone complications in sickle cell patients]. La Revue de Médecine Interne. 2022;**43**(8):479-486

[23] Lammert F, Gurusamy K, Ko CW, Miquel JF, Méndez-Sánchez N, Portincasa P, et al. Gallstones. Nature Reviews Disease Primers. 2016;**2**:16024

[24] Diehl AK, Sugarek NJ, Todd KH. Clinical evaluation for gallstone disease: usefulness of symptoms and signs in diagnosis. The American Journal of Medicine. 1990;**89**(1):29-33

[25] Minoli G, Imperiale G, Spinzi GC, Terruzzi V, Rigas B. Circadian periodicity and other clinical features of biliary pain. Journal of Clinical Gastroenterology. 1991;**13**(5):546-548

[26] Pereira SP, Veysey MJ, Kennedy C, Hussaini SH, Murphy GM, Dowling RH. Gallstone dissolution with oral bile acid therapy. Importance of pretreatment CT scanning and reasons for nonresponse. Digestive Diseases and Sciences. 1997;**42**(8):1775-1782

[27] Caroli A, Del Favero G, Di Mario F, Spigariol F, Scalon P, Meggiato T, et al. Computed tomography in predicting gall stone solubility: a prospective trial. Gut. 1992;**33**(5):698-700

[28] Shea JA, Berlin JA, Escarce JJ, Clarke JR, Kinosian BP, Cabana MD, et al. Revised estimates of diagnostic test sensitivity and specificity in suspected biliary tract disease. Archives of Internal Medicine. 1994;**154**(22):2573-2581

[29] Zakko SF, Srb S, Ramsby GR. Sensitivity of percutaneous endoscopy compared with ultrasonography in the detection of residue or mucosal lesions after topical gallbladder stone dissolution. Gastrointestinal Endoscopy. 1995;**42**(5):434-438

[30] Dahan P, Andant C, Lévy P, Amouyal P, Amouyal G, Dumont M, et al. Prospective evaluation of endoscopic ultrasonography and microscopic examination of duodenal bile in the diagnosis of cholecystolithiasis in 45

patients with normal conventional ultrasonography. Gut. 1996 Feb;**38**(2):277-281

[31] Tsai CJ, Leitzmann MF, Hu FB, Willett WC, Giovannucci EL. A prospective cohort study of nut consumption and the risk of gallstone disease in men. American Journal of Epidemiology. 2004;**160**(10):961-968

[32] Zhang YP, Li WQ, Sun YL, Zhu RT, Wang WJ. Systematic review with meta-analysis: coffee consumption and the risk of gallstone disease. Alimentary Pharmacology & Therapeutics. 2015;**42**(6):637-648

[33] European Association for the Study of the Liver (EASL). EASL Clinical Practice Guidelines on the prevention, diagnosis and treatment of gallstones. Journal of Hepatology. 2016;**65**(1):146-181

[34] Guarino MP, Cong P, Cicala M, Alloni R, Carotti S, Behar J. Ursodeoxycholic acid improves muscle contractility and inflammation in symptomatic gallbladders with cholesterol gallstones. Gut. 2007;**56**(6):815-820

[35] Walcher T, Haenle MM, Kron M, Hay B, Mason RA, Walcher D, et al. Vitamin C supplement use may protect against gallstones: an observational study on a randomly selected population. BMC Gastroenterology. 2009;**9**:74

[36] Gupta A, Gupta S, Siddeek RAT, Chennatt JJ, Singla T, Rajput D, et al. Demographic and clinicopathological profile of gall bladder cancer patients: study from a tertiary care center of the Sub-Himalayan region in Indo-Gangetic Belt. Journal of Carcinogenesis. 2021;**20**:6

[37] Schmidt MA, Marcano-Bonilla L, Roberts LR. Gallbladder cancer: epidemiology and genetic risk associations. Chinese Clinical Oncology. 2019;**8**(4):31

[38] Hyun JJ, Lee HS, Kim CD, Dong SH, Lee SO, Ryu JK, et al. Efficacy of magnesium trihydrate of ursodeoxycholic acid and chenodeoxycholic acid for gallstone dissolution: a prospective multicenter trial. Gut Liver. 2015;**9**(4):547-555

[39] Lee JM, Hyun JJ, Choi IY, Yeom SK, Kim SY, Jung SW, et al. Comparison on response and dissolution rates between ursodeoxycholic acid alone or in combination with chenodeoxycholic acid for gallstone dissolution according to stone density on CT scan: Strobe Compliant Observation Study. Medicine (Baltimore). 2015 Dec;**94**(50):e2037

[40] Petroni ML, Jazrawi RP, Pazzi P, et al. Ursodeoxycholic acid alone or with chenodeoxycholic acid for dissolution of cholesterol gallstones: a randomized multicentre trial. The British-Italian Gallstone Study Group. Alimentary Pharmacology & Therapeutics. 2001;**15**:123-128

[41] Senior JR, Johnson MF, DeTurck DM, Bazzoli F, Roda E. In vivo kinetics of radiolucent gallstone dissolution by oral dihydroxy bile acids. Gastroenterology. 1990;**99**(1):243-251

[42] Maton PN, Iser JH, Reuben A, Saxton HM, Murphy GM, Dowling RH. Outcome of chenodeoxycholic acid (CDCA) treatment in 125 patients with radiolucent gallstones. Factors influencing efficacy, withdrawal, symptoms and side effects and post-dissolution recurrence. Medicine (Baltimore). 1982;**61**(2):86-97

[43] Nagral S. Anatomy relevant to cholecystectomy. Journal of Minimal Access Surgery. 2005;**1**(2):53-58

[44] Pina LN, Samoilovich F, Urrutia S, Rodríguez A, Alle L, Ferreres AR. Surgical considerations of the cystic duct and heister valves. Surgery Journal (N Y). 2015;**1**(1):e23-e27

[45] Raghuwanshi DS, Ram M, Khan S, et al. Moynihan's hump: our eyes see what our mind knows. The Indian Journal of Surgery. 2021;**83**:1077-1078

[46] Hugh TB, Kelly MD, Mekisic A. Rouvière's sulcus: a useful landmark in laparoscopic cholecystectomy. The British Journal of Surgery. 1997;**84**(9):1253-1254

[47] Gupta V, Jain G. The R4U Planes for the zonal demarcation for safe laparoscopic cholecystectomy. World Journal of Surgery. 2021;**45**(4):1096-1101

[48] Strasberg SM, Hertl M, Soper NJ. An analysis of the problem of biliary injury during laparoscopic cholecystectomy. Journal of the American College of Surgeons. 1995;**180**(1):101-125

[49] Navarra G, Pozza E, Occhionorelli S, Carcoforo P, Donini I. One-wound laparoscopic cholecystectomy. The British Journal of Surgery. 1997;**84**:695

[50] Bhandarkar D, Mittal G, Shah R, Katara A, Udwadia TE. Single-incision laparoscopic cholecystectomy: how I do it? Journal of Minimal Access Surgery. 2011;**7**(1):17-23

[51] Pereira C, Gururaj S. A systematic review and meta-analysis of single-incision laparoscopic cholecystectomy versus conventional four-port laparoscopic cholecystectomy. Cureus. 2022;**14**(12):e32524

[52] Zorron R, Filgueiras M, Maggioni LC, et al. NOTES. Transvaginal cholecystectomy: report of the first case. Surgical Innovation. 2007;**14**:279-283

[53] Peng C, Ling Y, Ma C, Ma X, Fan W, Niu W, et al. Safety outcomes of NOTES cholecystectomy versus laparoscopic cholecystectomy: a systematic review and meta-analysis. Surgical Laparoscopy, Endoscopy & Percutaneous Techniques. 2016;**26**(5):347-353

[54] Shenoy R, Mederos MA, Ye L, et al. Intraoperative and postoperative outcomes of robot-assisted cholecystectomy: a systematic review. Systematic Reviews. 2021;**10**(1):124

Chapter 6

Gallbladder Cancer

Carlo de Werra, Antonio Vitiello, Roberto Peltrini, Biancamaria Iacone, Anna Tedesco, Antonio Coppola, Marcello Filotico, Bianca Pacilio and Antonio Gargiulo

Abstract

Gallbladder carcinoma is a form of cancer that develops in the gallbladder, an organ located beneath the liver. This condition poses a clinical challenge due to its late diagnosis and aggressive tumor behavior. Risk factors include the presence of gallstones, advanced age, and obesity. Diagnosis of gallbladder carcinoma requires the use of various diagnostic techniques such as ultrasound, computed tomography, and magnetic resonance imaging. Cholecystectomy, the surgical removal of the gallbladder, is the primary treatment for gallbladder carcinoma. However, management and treatment may require a multidisciplinary approach, which can also involve chemotherapy, radiation therapy, and targeted therapies. Increased awareness of this disease is necessary to improve early diagnosis and treatment options, ultimately enhancing survival rates and improving the quality of life for patients with gallbladder carcinoma.

Keywords: gallbladder, cancer, surgery, cholecystectomy, management, treatment

1. Introduction

Gallbladder cancer is a rare and highly aggressive malignancy that presents significant challenges for diagnosis and treatment [1]. Although it is a relatively uncommon cancer, its poor prognosis and the lack of effective treatments make it a significant concern for patients and healthcare providers alike [2]. Gallbladder cancer is often asymptomatic in its early stages, making it difficult to detect and diagnose [3]. Additionally, there are several risk factors associated with gallbladder cancer, including gallstones, chronic inflammation, obesity, and genetic factors, which further complicate the diagnostic process [1].

Treatment of gallbladder cancer typically involves surgery, but the extent of resection depends on the stage of the tumor [2]. Adjuvant therapies such as chemotherapy and radiation therapy have limited efficacy in the treatment of gallbladder cancer, but they may be used in select cases [3]. In this chapter, we will discuss the anatomy, pathogenesis, diagnosis, and treatment of gallbladder cancer, as well as its prognosis and follow-up care.

2. Anatomy

The gallbladder is a pear-shaped organ located on the underside of the liver in the right upper quadrant of the abdomen. It measures approximately 7–10 cm in length and 3–5 cm in diameter when fully distended [1]. The wall is thin with a thickness of 2–3 mm, and the mucosa has a simple columnar epithelium. Underneath, without a true submucosa, a single smooth muscle layer with longitudinal, circular, and oblique arrangement of fibers is observed.

The gallbladder is divided into three parts: the fundus, the body, and the neck (**Figure 1**). The fundus is the most distal portion of the gallbladder and projects beyond the inferior margin of the liver. The body of the gallbladder is in the midportion of the organ, while the neck is the narrowest portion of the gallbladder, which connects it to the cystic duct [4].

The gallbladder is supplied by the cystic artery, which is a branch of the right hepatic artery. The cystic vein drains into the portal vein. The gallbladder is innervated by the cystic nerve, which is a branch of the hepatic plexus. The cystic duct is the narrow tube that connects the gallbladder to the common bile duct, which carries bile from the liver to the small intestine [5].

The gallbladder functions as a storage and concentration reservoir for bile, a fluid produced by the liver that aids in the digestion and absorption of fats. When food enters the small intestine, the gallbladder contracts and releases stored bile into the duodenum via the common bile duct. The presence of gallstones, inflammation, or tumors in the gallbladder can disrupt this normal process and lead to various pathologies, including gallbladder cancer [1].

3. Pathophysiology and risk factors

For a long time, Cholangiocarcinoma (CC) has been regarded as an appropriate model for illustrating the relationship between chronic inflammation and cancer. In

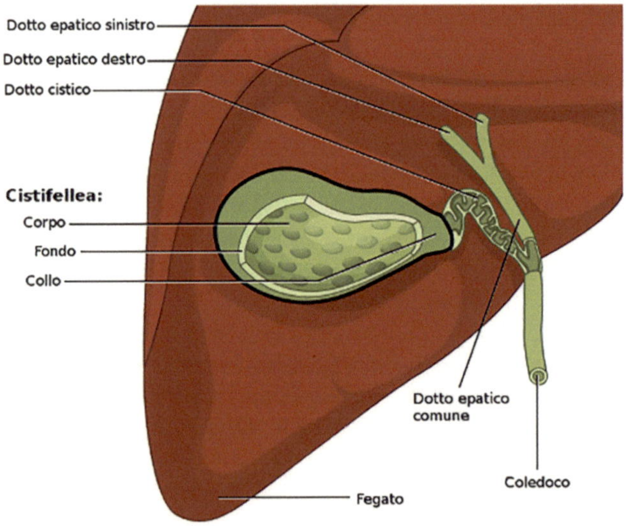

Figure 1.
Gallbladder anatomy.

1920, Archibald Leitch chose to study CC due to its association with a "...particular endogenous irritant," gallstones. He implanted human gallstones, pebbles, and tar pellets into the gallbladders of guinea pigs and observed a progressive worsening, starting from epithelial desquamation to lesions, and in some cases, the emergence of invasive adenocarcinomas [4]. He repeated the same experiment using melted lanolin, a soft material capable of causing repeated damage to cells, which did not, however, induce any macroscopic changes in the gallbladder. Leitch concluded that the damage was caused not by the nature of the irritant but by the mere presence of a foreign body, which was responsible for the development of a "[...] pathological state of the tissues" predisposing to the onset of cancer [6], the individual risk factors for gallbladder carcinoma:

- *Ethnicity*: It plays a colossal role in both the prevalence of gallbladder disease and the composition of gallstones. Cholesterol stones prevail in the Western world, while pigment stones are more common in Asia. Gallbladder cancer is rare in industrialized countries. In the United States, it accounts for 0.5% of gastrointestinal malignancies, with fewer than 5000 cases per year (1–2.5 cases per 100,000) [5]. Worldwide, gallbladder carcinoma has a low incidence, less than 2 cases per 100,000, although there is considerable variability. High incidence rates are found in Native Americans of North and South America, resulting in unusually high mortality rates, particularly among women. For example, in La Paz (Bolivia), the incidence is 15.5 per 100,000 in women (compared to 7.5 per 100,000 in men), and in New Mexico, it is 11.3 per 100,000 in women (compared to 4 per 100,000 in men). Furthermore, gallbladder carcinoma is one of the leading causes of cancer-related death in the female population of Chile, surpassing even breast, lung, and cervical cancer. In fact, it has been observed that in certain populations in North America (Native Americans of Western America and New Mexico), the incidence of gallbladder cancer is statistically higher (the annual incidence of gallbladder carcinoma per 100,000 individuals with gallstones is 74.9% in females of this race, with a range from 65.3 to 87.7%). Other regions at high risk include Eastern Europe (14 per 100,000 in Poland), northern India (21.5 per 100,000 in Delhi), and South Pakistan (11.3 per 100,000). An intermediate incidence risk (ranging from 3.7 to 9.1 per 100,000) is observed in Latin American populations, Israel (5 per 100,000), and Japan (7 per 100,000), related to the frequent congenital anatomical abnormalities associated with this cancer that are found in the Japanese population. Finally, areas where the frequency is increasing in recent years include Shanghai and China. These data also reflect the prevalence of cholelithiasis or Salmonella infections, which are highly prevalent in Indian populations in America.

- *Gender*: Gallbladder cancer exhibits a pronounced predilection for the female gender, especially in high-risk regions where the incidence among women reaches such remarkable heights that it warrants the appellation of "female gender bias." Females, particularly during the reproductive age, are twice as likely to develop gallstones. It is known that estrogens (endogenous or pharmacologically administered) increase the secretion of cholesterol into the bile. On the other hand, progesterone decreases the gallbladder's emptying capacity, promoting stasis [1].

- *Age*: The risk of developing gallbladder cancer escalates concomitantly with advancing age, with the highest morbidity rates observed within the age range of 50–60 years (encompassing 80–90% of all gallbladder carcinoma cases). This compelling data holds immense significance when juxtaposed with the equally noteworthy prevalence of gallstone disease in women, which manifests approximately a decade earlier within a relatively younger age cohort [3]. The type of stones also varies depending on the age group: younger patients mostly have cholesterol stones (due to bile oversaturation), while older individuals have a higher incidence of pigment stones. Additionally, age is a factor that increases the risk of complications, emphasizing the crucial role of preventive cholecystectomy.

- *Chronic inflammation*: Intriguing studies reveal that approximately 25% of cases manifest a fascinating phenomenon known as the porcelain gallbladder, although recent research endeavors have cast doubt upon this observation. Remarkably, it seems that only gallbladders showcasing partial calcifications or multiple punctate calcifications precisely nestled within the glandular expanse of the mucosa are to be considered as true premalignant conditions, warranting proactive removal as a preventive measure. In addition, the persistent presence of chronic bacterial infections fervently fuels gallbladder irritation and inflammation, adding another layer of complexity to the intricate puzzle. Notably, carriers of the notorious S. Typhi bacterium face an astonishingly heightened risk, spanning an alarming 8 to 12-fold increase of eventually succumbing to the treacherous grips of carcinoma [4]. Meanwhile, the cunning culprit H. pylori emerges as an insidious player, with an odds ratio of 6.5 in the Japanese population and an equally compelling ratio of 5.86 in their Thai counterparts, perpetuating the bewildering web of gallbladder cancer causation. Furthermore, the intriguing realm of primary sclerosing cholangitis (PSC) unfurls an intriguing association, with a staggering 37% of cases exhibiting coexisting dysplasia while 14% plunge into the abyss of adenocarcinoma.

- *Congenital anomalies of the biliary tract*: Unveiling their prominence predominantly within the Asian populace, these captivating aberrations encompass the enigmatic domain of pancreaticobiliary junctional irregularities. Within this captivating tapestry, the prophylactic act of cholecystectomy assumes paramount significance, acting as a robust shield against the looming specter of gallbladder cancer that hauntingly pervades the afflicted individuals with exceptional frequency [5].

- *Gallbladder polyps*: Within the enigmatic realm of the gallbladder, a captivating subplot emerges—polyps. These elusive entities captivate our attention, affecting 5% of adults, often masquerading as potential harbingers of gallbladder malignancy. However, amidst this intricate tapestry, most gallbladder polyps gracefully assume the role of benign cholesterol lesions or fibromyoglandular growths, devoid of malicious intent. Yet, lurking within this benign facade, true papillary neoplasms (formerly known as adenomas) may conceal their treacherous potential, their virulence intricately linked to their voluminous presence and flourishing vascularity. As we delve deeper into this captivating narrative, a remarkable revelation surfaces—polyps with a diameter less than 1cm seldom harbor sinister aspirations, assuring a semblance of respite. However, as the stage expands, embracing polyps exceeding the 2 cm threshold, a tantalizing secret reveals itself, their bosom potentially concealing malignant neoplasms. Thus, a symphony of data illuminates our path, emphasizing a heightened incidence of cancer in polyps boasting a diameter surpassing the majestic 1 cm mark and those adorned with a delicate vascular pedicle [7, 8]

- *Gallbladder stones*: Unveiling the intricate interplay between gallbladder cancer and its stony companions, the enigmatic saga of cholelithiasis unfolds. A compelling tale emerges as a positive history of gallstone affliction casts a shadow of elevated risk, with a resolute relative risk of 4.9. It is a realm where dualities coexist, where the majority (ranging from 69 to 100%) of gallbladder cancer warriors share a clandestine bond with gallstones, though not every warrior bears this emblem. Yet, within the fabric of this entwined narrative, a symphony of coexistence resonates, whispering of gallstones assuming the enigmatic role of co-factors, propelling the genesis of gallbladder carcinoma. A poignant revelation surfaces, shining a radiant light upon Native Americans, adorned with an abundance of cholesterol stones, who, in their unique tapestry, bear witness to an amplified incidence of gallbladder cancer [7]. As we traverse this intricate labyrinth, dimensions assume significance—size expands beyond mere physicality, transcending the 3 cm threshold, accompanied by an army of brethren, numbers and weight, their presence inextricably linked to an escalated risk of cancer. Yet, amidst this grand stage, the passage of time assumes a lesser role, its duration holding a diminished sway. Within the realm of gallstone- laden warriors battling cancer, a dichotomy of stone composition unfolds—cholesterol stones proudly claim their dominion, while pigment stones grace the stage with a more subdued presence. Inextricably intertwined, the veil of cancer incidence lifts, exposing the profound impact of cholecystectomies, their dwindling numbers invoking a crescendo of carcinogenic potential. Beyond the realm of cholesterol, the shadows of bile's carcinogenicity come to light—bile acids (cholic acid, chenodeoxycholic acid, deoxycholic acid, ursodeoxycholic acid, and lithocholic acid), whether tethered to conjugates or roaming free, dance amidst the population mosaic, unveiling their disparate distribution. Within the realm of gallstone warriors, striding alongside their cancerous comrades, a revelation emerges—an ethereal surge of deconjugated lithocholic acid, reaching crescendos of tumorigenicity, weaving the intricate threads of endogenous carcinogenesis within the gallbladder's realm. As we delve deeper into this captivating narrative, an array of factors intertwined with gallstone formation springs forth, further illuminating the complex tapestry that weaves the tale of gallbladder affliction [8, 9]

- *Family history and genetics*: Genetic susceptibility is a key factor in stone formation, which is a stepwise process regulated by numerous genes. Among the better-known genes are apolipoprotein E (APOE) and B (APOB), cholesterol ester transfer protein (CEPT), cholesterol 7-alpha-hydroxylase, cholecystokinin A receptor (CCAR), and LDL receptor (LDLR). The spotlight shines brightly on the apolipoprotein B (APOB) gene, standing alone as the unequivocally identified culprit in gallbladder carcinogenesis [9].

The gene most recently associated with stone formation and predisposition to gallbladder cancer is ABCG8, which encodes a cholesterol transporter present on the canalicular membrane of hepatocytes. However, it is important to note that cholelithiasis is a polygenic disease with a complex etiology.

- *Obesity and metabolic syndrome/dyslipidemia/diabetes mellitus*: Obesity, especially central (visceral) obesity, is a well-known risk factor for gallbladder disease. One in four obese individuals suffers from gallstones. Individuals with dyslipidemia (low levels of HDL, high levels of triglycerides) also have an increased risk of stone formation. These two conditions (central obesity and dyslipidemia), along with fasting hyperglycemia and hypertension, are part of Metabolic Syndrome. One of the most plausible mechanisms involves the enhancing role of high insulin levels (resulting from insulin resistance) on cholesterol transporters in hepatocytes.

- *Rapid weight loss*: A hypocaloric diet leading to a weight loss of more than 1kg per week significantly increases the risk of gallstone formation. This condition is frequently observed during the first 6 weeks of follow-up in severely obese individuals undergoing bariatric surgery.

- *Total parenteral nutrition (TPN)*: TPN is a well-known risk factor for the formation of sludge or biliary sludge. After approximately 5–10 days of intensive TPN therapy, sludge formation is common, reaching a prevalence of 50% if TPN is extended to 30 days and 100% for therapies lasting more than 6 weeks. This condition occurs due to the cessation of enteric stimulation on the gallbladder and the resulting biliary stasis.

- *Other associated conditions*: Pathologies associated with the development of gallstones include cirrhosis, hepatitis C, non-alcoholic fatty liver disease, sickle cell anemia, Crohn's disease, and cystic fibrosis. In the latter two conditions, malabsorption leads to depletion of total bile salts and indirect cholesterol supersaturation in the bile.

- *Other lifestyle factors*: Other risk factors include cigarette smoking and alcohol consumption (in men only) [8].

From a genetic perspective, the polymorphism of the ABCG8-DH19 partner gene, ABCG5/G8, was the first discovered genetic risk factor for the formation of cholesterol gallstones [10]. This lithogenic polymorphism leads to a gain of function in the protein, allowing for increased biliary secretion of cholesterol on the canalicular side of hepatocyte membrane, contributing to bile supersaturation and promoting stone formation [11]. Interestingly, in addition to its role as a risk factor for gallstone formation, this polymorphism has also been associated with an increased risk of developing gallbladder cancer in different ethnicities [12, 13].

Furthermore, polymorphisms of genes related to the immune system, inflammation, and oxidative stress have been associated with an increased risk of gallbladder cancer. These genes include PTGS2 [14], TLR2, TLR4 [15], IL1RN, IL1B [16], IL10 [17], IL8 [18], CCR5 [19], LXRβ [20], and OGG1 [21].

Studies in murine models have shown that mice with cholesterol microstones (early stage of gallstone formation) exhibited a gallbladder characterized by increased mucosal layer thickness and elevated interleukin-1 and myeloperoxidase activity in the gallbladder wall [22]. Morphological changes (epithelial hyperplasia, hypertrophic muscularis propria, and increased wall thickness) were observed as early as four weeks. These changes were accompanied by an inflammatory infiltrate composed of eosinophils, macrophages, neutrophils, and lymphocytes within the lamina propria [23]. At this point, Maurer et al. demonstrated that T lymphocytes are crucial for the development of cholesterol gallstones, as Rag2 -/- mice lacking T and B lymphocytes were resistant to cholesterol gallstone formation despite being fed a lithogenic diet for 8 weeks [24]. This showed that, at least in murine models of cholelithiasis, chronic inflammation of the gallbladder occurs in the early stages of lithogenesis as a local response to the presence of cholesterol supersaturation in bile even before the formation of macroscopic gallstones [25].

Gallstones, along with the associated cholecystitis, lead to a sequence of events that result in dysplasia and eventually carcinoma of the gallbladder in over 90% of cases. This assertion is supported by the fact that 83% of gallbladders with stones are associated with inflammation, showing at least one focus of hyperplasia, while 13.5% exhibit atypical hyperplasia and 3.5% show carcinoma in situ.

Two patterns of malignant transformation have been observed in the gallbladder: the metaplasia- dysplasia-carcinoma sequence (**Figure 2**) and the adenoma-carcinoma sequence. However, carcinogenesis related to biliary lithiasis primarily occurs through the metaplasia-dysplasia- carcinoma pathway, rather than transformation from a pre-existing benign tumor lesion.

Metaplasia is a common finding in gallbladder tissues exposed to gallstones, with frequencies ranging from 59.5 to 95.0% for pseudopyloric metaplasia and 9.5–58.1% for intestinal metaplasia [26, 27]. Furthermore, the severity of lesions found in the epithelium worsens with increasing weight, volume (particularly if it is > 3 cm), and variation in the shape of gallstones (spherical shape being less injurious) [28].

Moreover, metaplastic lesions arise under the expression of key transcription factors that redirect the epithelial phenotype to a different type. In fact, gallbladder metaplasia is often associated with the expression of CDX2 [29], a homeobox transcription factor involved in the normal development of the intestine, commonly found in intestinal metaplasia of the esophagus and stomach as well [30]. The normal epithelium of the gallbladder does not express CDX2, and the surrounding leukocytes

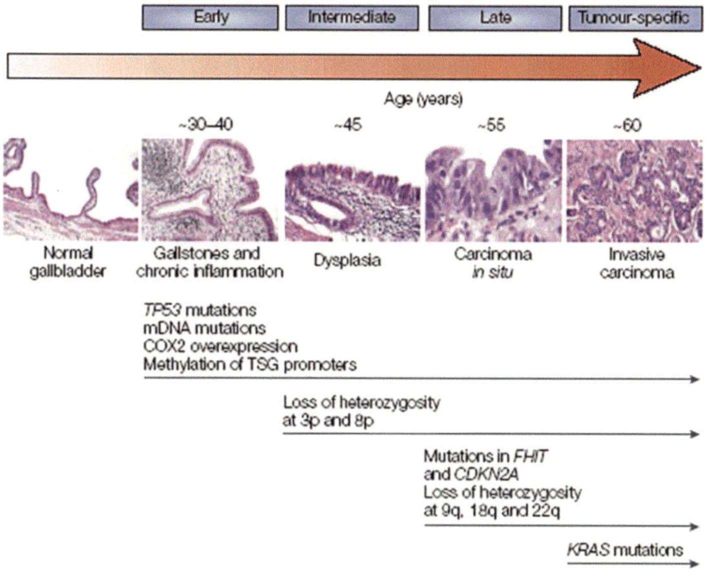

Figure 2.
Progression of gallbladder cancer.

mainly consist of T lymphocytes (CD3+, CD4+, and CD8+) and populations of macrophages (CD14+, CD68+, and CD163+), with low or absent levels of B cells (CD20+). In contrast, the CDX2-positive metaplastic epithelium of the gallbladder is often infiltrated by dense populations of T cells, B cells, and macrophages.

Furthermore, the presence of metaplastic changes is correlated with an increase in the average thickness of the gallbladder wall. Diffuse thickening of the gallbladder wall, defined as an enlargement exceeding 3 mm measured on ultrasound examination, can be observed in primary inflammatory processes, such as acute, chronic, and acalculous cholecystitis.

Certain types of infections, likely due to bile and bile salt deconjugation, can also contribute to the development of gallbladder cancer (infection by Salmonella typhi, Clonorchis sinensis, Opisthorchis viverrini, as well as various species of Escherichia, Klebsiella, and Helicobacter) [31]. Although little is known about the true carcinogenic effect of Salmonella in the absence of gallstones, there is consistent epidemiological evidence that chronic Salmonella infection is a risk factor for gallbladder cancer. It is known that Salmonella infection is even more potent in this regard when gallstones are present. Both gallstones and bacteria can induce an inflammatory response, so it is plausible to hypothesize that the combination of these agents increases the risk of developing gallbladder cancer.

Reflux of pancreatic juice into the bile ducts and the gallbladder itself can underlie the development of gallbladder carcinoma, as supported by experimental findings that have shown a higher incidence of this disease in individuals with anomalous drainage of the Wirsung and common bile duct into the duodenum (Anomalous arrangement of the pancreaticobiliary duct AAPBD) [32]. These patients exhibited an extramural common segment of the two ducts, i.e., an extrasphincteric portion (evaluated by cholangiography), which allowed reflux of pancreatic juice into the bile duct. AAPBD is a congenital biliary anomaly associated with a high frequency of gallbladder carcinoma, with relative risks ranging from 167.2 to 419.6 times higher in AAPBD patients compared to the general population [33]. In these patients, carcinogenesis progresses through a sequence of metaplasia- dysplasia-carcinoma driven by chronic inflammation, like gallbladder cancer caused by gallstones. Under the influence of this chronic inflammation, activation of pancreatic enzymes, changes in the bile acid fraction, and production of mutagenic or occasionally carcinogenic substances may occur [34]. It is interesting to note that the prevalence of KRAS mutations is higher in AAPBD-related gallbladder cancer compared to non-related cases [35, 36], making it more etiologically like pancreatic cancer (which has a high prevalence of KRAS mutations) than LB-associated gallbladder cancer (where the frequency of such rearrangement is low or nonexistent). Generally, cancer associated with anomalous pancreaticobiliary ductal junction (APBDJ) occurs at a young age and is less correlated with female gender and cholelithiasis.

Some diseases are commonly associated with the development of gallbladder cancer è [37]. One of these is "porcelain" gallbladder, although recent studies do not support this correlation, although they still recommend gallbladder removal due to the associated symptoms, which are also difficult to diagnose preoperatively [38]. Adenomatous polyps have always been associated with a high risk of cancer when they exceed 10 mm in size, but neoplastic polyps can also be smaller, so careful long- term follow-up is necessary to avoid setting a criterion that is too permissive. Malignancy characteristics of polyps are determined by their irregular and heterogeneous echotexture, generally isoechoic with the liver, or hypoechoic, as well as by thickening of the gallbladder walls. In general, 3–8% of polyps are malignant, regardless of size (0–5% if <10 mm) [39]. Furthermore, certain autoimmune diseases have been associated with an increased risk of tumors [40], including gallbladder cancer [41]. Recently, six autoimmune conditions have been correlated with higher standardized incidence rates for gallbladder cancer: primary sclerosing cholangitis (PSC), celiac disease, Crohn's disease, pernicious anemia, ulcerative colitis, and polymyositis/dermatomyositis. PSC is the classic hepatobiliary manifestation of inflammatory bowel diseases and other immunomediated diseases, characterized by bile duct destruction and progression to end-stage liver disease. Chronic lesions occur in small, medium, and large bile ducts with inflammatory and obliterative concentric periductal fibrosis, leading to biliary stenosis. Metaplasia, dysplasia, and carcinoma of the gallbladder occur with high frequency in patients with PSC. The metaplasia-displasia-carcinoma sequence observed in the context of PSC is like that proposed for sporadic gallbladder cancer. In a histological study of 72 resected gallbladders in patients with PSC, significant morphological alterations were found: lymphoplasmacytic chronic cholecystitis was present in 49%, pseudopyloric metaplasia in 96%, intestinal metaplasia in 50%, dysplasia in 37%, and adenocarcinoma in 14% of the samples. The close association between gallbladder neoplasia and intrahepatic bile duct neoplasms supports the concept of "field cancerization" in the biliary tract of patients with PSC. Approximately half of patients with PSC have gallbladder abnormalities, and about 25% have stones in the bile duct. In another series of 102 patients with PSC who underwent cholecystectomy, 13% had a gallbladder neoplasm, and of these, 7% had adenocarcinoma and 6% had a benign tumor [42]. As exemplified by PSC, autoimmune diseases likely increase the risk of gallbladder cancer through the exacerbation of biliary inflammation.

4. Diagnosis

Ultrasonography (US) is the first-line approach and a valuable screening tool in patients with gallstone disease, which is known to be the primary risk factor for gallbladder cancer (**Figure 3**) [43–47]. However, it has several limitations: (1) it cannot fully stage the tumor, as it does not accurately visualize lymph nodes, peritoneal extension, and distant metastases; (2) it lacks pathognomonic signs, especially in early stages where nonspecific wall thickening can be indistinguishable from adenomyomatosis or chronic cholecystitis, particularly if extensive, considering that gallbladder cancer tends to cause localized thickening [48].

The evaluation of carcinoembryonic antigen (CEA) has shown utility in the diagnosis of gallbladder cancer. Recent studies have identified three types of glycoproteins (I, II, and III) in the biliary tract, with type I being present in normal epithelium. In cases of chronic inflammatory lesions, glycoprotein I is replaced by types II and III, with the latter being immunologically identical to CEA. However, these results lack statistical significance and cannot be considered useful for early diagnosis [49, 50].

Contrast-enhanced Computed Tomography (CT) has a diagnostic capability for detecting gallbladder tumors with a sensitivity of 88%, specificity of 87%, and overall diagnostic accuracy of 87%. The main indication for using CT in gallbladder cancer is staging, as this modality can demonstrate neoplastic extension to the gallbladder bed and the surrounding liver (in 60% of cases), as well as the presence of regional lymph node metastases, peritoneal metastases, and distant metastases (**Figure 4**). Angio- CT assesses the degree of vascular infiltration in the portal vein or hepatic artery, which is

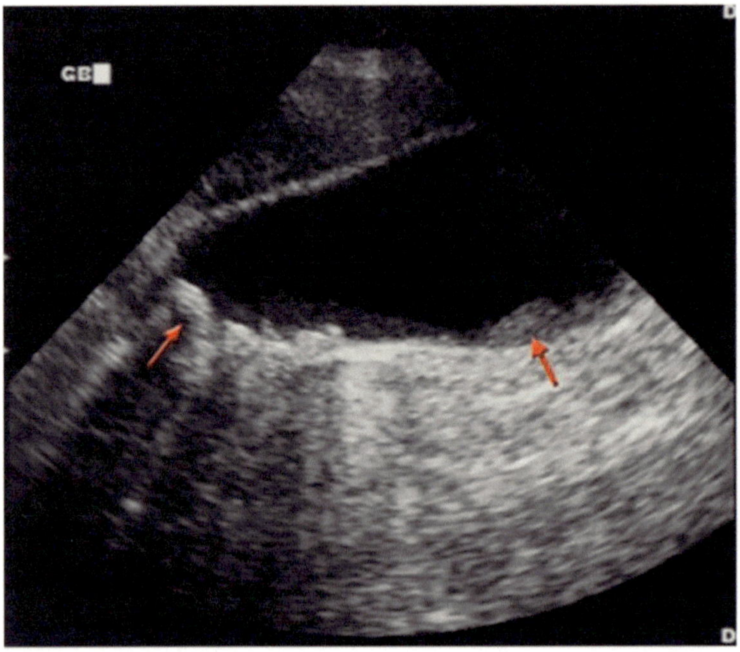

Figure 3.
US: Gallbladder adenocarcinoma.

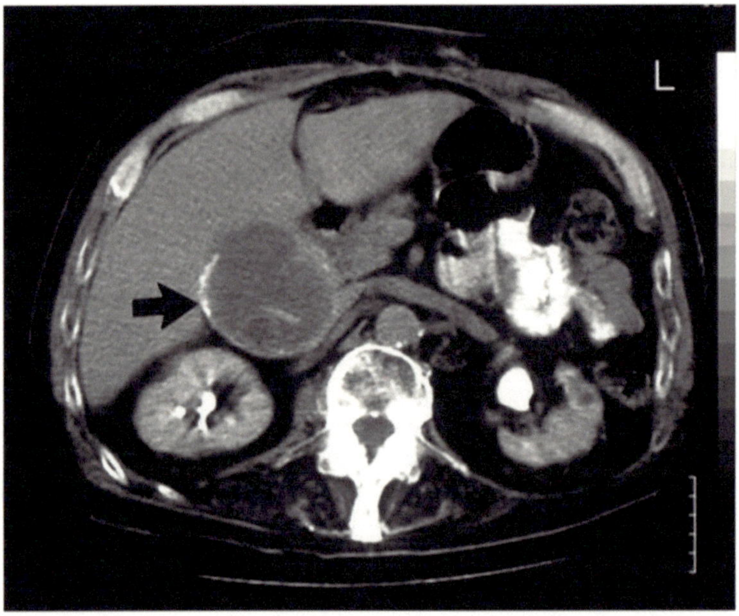

Figure 4.
CT: Gallbladder carcinoma with thickened walls capturing contrast medium.

important for preoperative evaluation. Differential diagnosis with xanthogranulomatous cholecystitis poses challenges due to overlapping features such as gallbladder wall thickening, involvement of adjacent organs including pericholecystic adipose tissue, portal lymph nodes, and the liver. In the diagnosis of gallbladder cancer, differential diagnosis and determination of local tumor extent are crucial. For these purposes, imaging techniques such as Endoscopic Ultrasound (EUS), CT, Magnetic Resonance Imaging (MRI), and Magnetic Resonance Cholangiopancreatography (MRCP) are useful.

Endoscopic Ultrasound (EUS) has a good sensitivity (92–97%) in differentiating gallbladder cancer from benign conditions [51, 52].

MRI is not a commonly used imaging modality in the diagnostic workup of gallbladder cancer; however, it can provide useful information [53–55].

MRCP can provide information on the infiltration of the main bile duct and the extent of intracholecystic tumor.

Positron Emission Tomography with Fluorodeoxyglucose (PET-FDG) can be considered as a complementary examination for the detection of non-abdominal metastases, guiding the surgeon towards radical re-intervention [56, 57].

Another valuable diagnostic tool is ultrasound-guided Fine-Needle Aspiration Biopsy (FNAB), which is accurate, rapid, and cost-effective. Unfortunately, gallbladder cancer has a high potential for dissemination, and the risk of tumor seeding along the needle tract is elevated. Laparoscopic experience with incidental gallbladder cancers has confirmed this risk, with reported cases of tumor implantation along trocar tracks or through the umbilicus during gallbladder extraction. Therefore, the answer is clear: biopsy should not be performed. In cases of uncertainty regarding both the nature of the neoplasm and its potential resectability (10–15% of cases), laparoscopic visualization and a supporting trocar allow, in almost all cases, a definitive assessment of the feasibility of radical surgery.

Currently, in the absence of preoperative diagnosis, an extensive intraoperative core needle biopsy with immediate analysis of frozen sections is preferred before initiating radical resection. In cases where granulomatous cholecystitis is frequently present with large calculi and extensive inflammation, limiting the possibility of a simple cholecystectomy, it is advisable to perform cholecystectomy with stone removal only after intraoperative biopsy has confirmed the absence of malignant neoplasms [58].

Finally, regarding laparoscopy, it can be confidently stated that it represents an excellent diagnostic tool for closed abdomen gallbladder cancer. Despite the era of significant technological advancements in diagnostic imaging, there are suggestive signs of neoplasms that can sometimes only be detected through laparoscopic exploration.

5. Staging

To stage gallbladder cancer, various classification systems can be used, all considering the most relevant prognostic factors: tumor type, size, depth of wall infiltration, invasion of adjacent organs, and metastatic spread via blood vessels, lymphatic system, and peritoneum.

The staging system of the Japanese Biliary Surgical Society divides tumors into 4 stages:

Stage 1: Cancer confined to the gallbladder capsule.

Stage 2: Cancer with lymph node involvement (N1) and/or minimal invasion of the liver/bile ducts.

Stage 3: Lymph node involvement (N2) and/or significant invasion of the liver/bile ducts.

Stage 4: Presence of distant metastases.

The Nevin classification is widely accepted in the Western world. It considers the stage of the neoplasm and the degree of cellular differentiation. In addition to its diagnostic significance, it also has prognostic value and provides therapeutic guidance by formulating tables with combined numbers for stage and grade. Nevin reported a 5-year survival rate of 21% after cholecystectomy in patients at stages I (intramucosal cancer or carcinoma in situ) and II (invasion of the mucosa and muscular layer), contrasting with poor outcomes in stages III (full-thickness invasion), IV (presence of metastasis in pericystic lymph nodes), and V (hepatic invasion and/or distant metastasis). Donohue et al. modified the Nevin system to include tumors involving the liver adjacent to the gallbladder in stage III and non-adjacent tumors in stage V [59, 60].

However, to date, the most well-known and widely used classification is undoubtedly the TNM classification (**Table 1**) [61].

Regarding histopathological grading, we distinguish:

- G1, well-differentiated carcinoma
- G2, moderately differentiated carcinoma
- G3, poorly differentiated carcinoma
- G4, undifferentiated carcinoma.

The AJCC/UICC staging is based precisely on the TNM classification [62]. The main conceptual difference with the Nevin classification is that the latter does not differentiate tumors that invade the muscular layer without invading the liver and does

Stage	T category	N category	M category	Estimated 5-year survival (%)
0	Tis	N0	M0	80–100
I	T1a (lamina propria)	N0	M0	80–100
	T1b (muscularis)	N0	M0	80–100
II	T2a (peritoneal side)	N0	M0	40–75
	T2b (hepatic side)	N0	M0	28–50
IIIa	T3	N0	M0	8–28
IIIb	T1, T2, T3	N1	M0	8
IVa	T4	N0, N1	M0	7
IVb	Any T	N2	M0	4
	Any T	Any N	M1	0–2

Source: References [2, 42].
**AJCC = American Joint Committee on Cancer.*

Table 1.
TNM staging according to the Eighth Edition of the AJCC Manual.*

not make a distinction based on tumor size. These two characteristics have significant prognostic significance. Partial or total invasion of the muscular layer is essential considering that the lymphatic drainage of the gallbladder lies between the muscular layer and the serosa. The pre-muscular subserosa is a plane composed of connective tissue, nerve endings, blood vessels, lymphatics, and adipocytes; it is not covered by the serosa in the portion of the gallbladder that is nestled in the liver, but it represents a key element for neoplastic dissemination, considering that in most cholecystectomies for cholelithiasis, the subserosal plane is the easiest for dissection. In incidental tumors that have invaded the muscular layer, this allows an open pathway for tumor metastasis through the lymphatic route [59].

6. Treatment

Gallbladder cancer treatment depends on several factors, such as the stage of cancer, overall health, and patient's preference [63]. Surgical resection is the primary treatment for localized gallbladder cancer, which involves removing the gallbladder, surrounding lymph nodes, and portions of the liver and bile ducts [64]. A radical cholecystectomy is generally recommended, but a laparoscopic cholecystectomy may be appropriate for select patients with early-stage cancer who have no invasion into surrounding tissues [65].

For patients with advanced or metastatic disease, a multidisciplinary approach is necessary, which may include systemic chemotherapy, radiation therapy, or a combination of these modalities [66]. Chemotherapy regimens for gallbladder cancer may include gemcitabine and cisplatin, or other combinations of cytotoxic agents [67]. The use of immunotherapy, such as immune checkpoint inhibitors, has shown promise in early clinical trials but requires further research to understand the role in the treatment of gallbladder cancer [68]. Palliative measures, such as biliary stenting, pain management, and nutritional support, may also be used to manage symptoms and improve quality of life for patients with advanced gallbladder cancer [64].

The surgical management of gallbladder cancer depends on several factors, including the extent and location of the tumor, the patient's overall health status, and the experience of the surgeon [64]. Surgical removal of the gallbladder (cholecystectomy) is the primary treatment option for early- stage gallbladder cancer that is confined to the gallbladder and has not spread to nearby lymph nodes or organs [65]. Laparoscopic (**Figure 5**) or robotic-assisted cholecystectomy is associated with less pain, shorter hospital stays, and faster recovery times compared to open surgery [69].

For more advanced gallbladder cancer, surgery may involve removal of the gallbladder, portions of the liver, and nearby lymph nodes. This is known as a radical cholecystectomy and may be done using an open or minimally invasive approach (**Figure 6**) [64].

Despite the challenges, surgical management remains the most effective treatment option for localized gallbladder cancer, and advances in surgical techniques, systemic therapies, and supportive care have improved outcomes for patients [70]. The success of surgery depends on several factors, including the stage of the cancer, the experience of the surgical team, and the patient's overall health status [64]. The treatment of gallbladder cancer requires a multidisciplinary approach, with close collaboration between surgeons, medical oncologists, radiation oncologists, and other specialists [66]. The goal of treatment is to maximize the chances of cure while minimizing treatment-related side effects and optimizing quality of life for the patient [70].

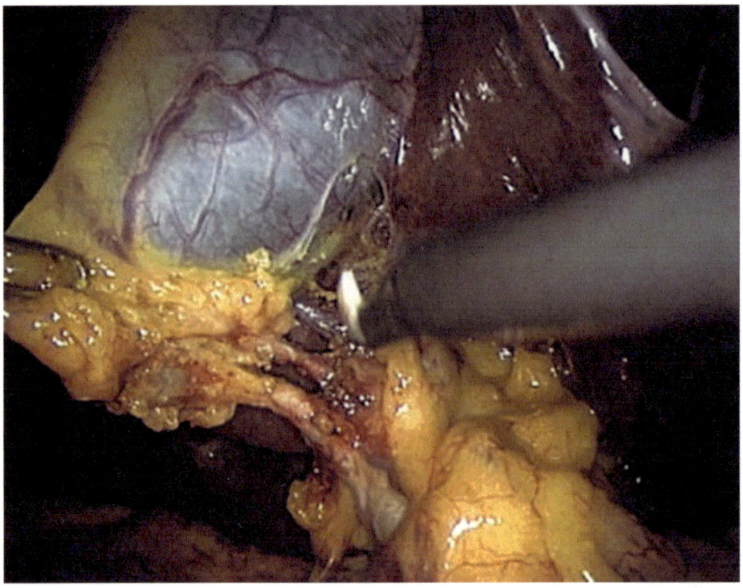

Figure 5.
VLS colecystectomy.

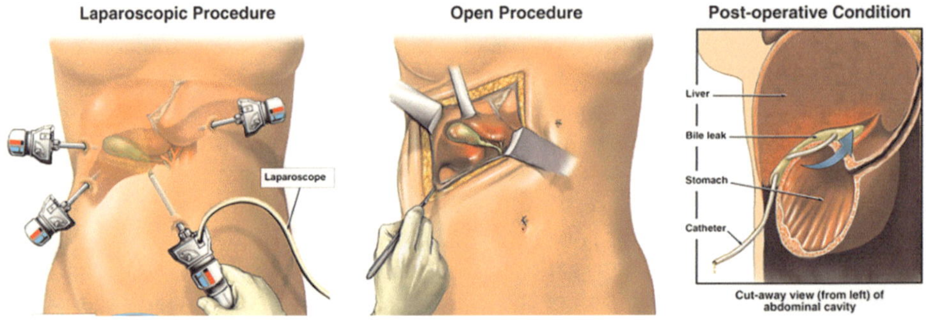

Figure 6.
Laparoscopic vs open procedure.

7. Prognosis and follow-up

The prognosis for gallbladder cancer varies depending on the stage of the cancer at diagnosis, with earlier stage cancers having a better prognosis than more advanced stage cancers. Other factors that can impact prognosis include the size and location of the tumor, the patient's overall health status, and the presence of other medical conditions [1].

For patients with early-stage gallbladder cancer that has not spread beyond the gallbladder, the five-year survival rate is around 80%. However, for patients with more advanced stage cancer that has spread to nearby organs or lymph nodes, the five-year survival rate is much lower, around 5–10% [2].

In chronic carriers of large gallstones, the best prevention for gallbladder cancer is cholecystectomy, as shown in a case-control study of 81 patients in 1983 by Andrew K. Diehl.

After surgery, patients with gallbladder cancer will require close monitoring to detect any signs of recurrence. This may involve regular imaging tests, such as CT scans or ultrasounds, as well as blood tests to monitor for tumor markers. The frequency and duration of follow-up will depend on the stage of the cancer, the patient's overall health status, and other factors [1].

In addition to imaging and blood tests, follow-up for gallbladder cancer may also involve monitoring for symptoms such as jaundice, abdominal pain, and weight loss, which may indicate recurrence or metastasis. Patients should also be counseled on lifestyle modifications, such as maintaining a healthy diet and exercise routine, and avoiding tobacco and excessive alcohol consumption, to help reduce the risk of recurrence [71].

In cases where the cancer has spread beyond the gallbladder, additional treatments such as chemotherapy, radiation therapy, or targeted therapy may be recommended. These treatments may be used before or after surgery, depending on the specific circumstances of the patient's case [1].

Overall, the prognosis for gallbladder cancer can be challenging, particularly in cases where the cancer has already spread beyond the gallbladder. However, with appropriate treatment and close follow-up, many patients can achieve good outcomes and maintain a good quality of life [2].

8. Conclusions

In conclusion, gallbladder cancer is a rare but serious malignancy that presents many challenges for patients and healthcare providers. Early detection is key to improving outcomes, and surgical resection remains the mainstay of treatment for most patients. However, the complex anatomy and physiology of the gallbladder and biliary system can make surgical management of gallbladder cancer difficult, requiring specialized expertise and careful planning [1].

Despite these challenges, recent advances in diagnostic and imaging technologies, as well as in surgical and non-surgical treatment options, offer hope for patients with gallbladder cancer. With ongoing research and improved understanding of the pathogenesis and molecular biology of this disease, new targeted therapies and personalized treatment approaches may become available in the future [2].

In the meantime, it is important for patients with gallbladder cancer to receive multidisciplinary care from a team of experienced healthcare providers, including surgeons, oncologists, radiologists, and other specialists as needed. Through collaboration and a patient-centered approach to care, we can continue to make progress in the fight against gallbladder cancer and improve outcomes for patients [1].

Author details

Carlo de Werra[1*], Antonio Vitiello[2], Roberto Peltrini[2], Biancamaria Iacone[2], Anna Tedesco[2], Antonio Coppola[1], Marcello Filotico[3], Bianca Pacilio[1] and Antonio Gargiulo[2]

1 General, Endocrine, Metabolic, and Bariatric Surgery Complex Operative Unit, University of Naples Federico II, Naples, Italy

2 General, Oncological and Minimally Invasive Surgery Complex Operative Unit, University of Naples Federico II, Naples, Italy

3 Department of Advanced Biomedical Sciences, University of Naples Federico II, Naples, Italy

*Address all correspondence to: dewerra@unina.it

References

[1] Hundal R, Shaffer EA, Gallinger S. Diagnosis and management of gallbladder cancer: A review. Journal of Surgical Oncology. 2014;**110**(5):572-581

[2] Liu X, Wang Y, Li Y, Sun X, Qi Y, Zhang Y. Current status and challenges of early diagnosis and treatment of gallbladder cancer. World Journal of Gastrointestinal Oncology. 2019;**11**(11):1067-1084

[3] Waseem D, Tushar T, Harrison S. Gallbladder Cancer. StatPearls Publishing; 2020

[4] Roskott AM, Chauhan SS, Hasan SA. Gallbladder Anatomy. StatPearls Publishing; 2020

[5] Memis A, Kantarci F, Incebiyik A, Ozturk G. Evaluation of the cystic duct and its variations with magnetic resonance cholangiography. Journal of Clinical Imaging Science. 2019;**9**:20

[6] Leitch A. A British Medical Association lecture on gallstones and cancer of the gallbladder: An Experimental Study. British Medical Journal. 1924;**2**:451-454

[7] Aloia TA et al. Gallbladder cancer: Expert consensus statement. H.P.B. 2015;**17**(8):661-744

[8] Espinoza JA et al. The inflammatory inception of gallbladder cancer. Biochimica et Biophysica Acta (BBA)—Reviews on Cancer. 2016;**1865**(2):245-254

[9] Zhou L et al. Expression of LAPTM4B in gallbladder carcinoma cells: The role in invasive potential. Hepatogastroenterology. 2014;**57**(98):207-21154

[10] Krawczyk M, Wang DQ, Portincasa P, Lammert F. Dissecting the genetic heterogeneityof gallbladder stone formation. Seminars in Liver Disease. 2011;**31**:157-172

[11] Von Kampen O. Genetic and functional identification of the likely causative variant for cholesterol gallstone disease at the ABCG5/8 lithogenic locus. Hepatology. 2013;**57**:2407-2417

[12] Xu HL et al. Cholesterol metabolism gene polymorphisms and the risk of biliary tract cancers and stones: A population-based case–control study in Shanghai. China Carcinogen. 2011;**32**:58-62

[13] Srivastava A et al. Single nucleotide polymorphism in the ABCG8 transporter gene is associated with gallbladder cancer susceptibility. Liver International. 2009;**29**:831-837

[14] Srivastava K et al. Functional polymorphisms of the cyclooxygenase (PTGS2) gene and risk for gallbladder cancer in a North Indian population. Journal of Gastroenterology. 2009;**44**:774-780

[15] Srivastava K et al. Significant association between toll-like receptor gene polymorphisms and gallbladder cancer. Liver International. 2010;**30**:1067-1072

[16] Vishnoi M et al. IL-1 gene polymorphisms and genetic susceptibility of gallbladder cancer in a north Indian population. Cancer Genetics and Cytogenetics. 2008;**186**:63-68

[17] Hsing AW et al. Variants in inflammation genes and the risk of

biliary tract cancers and stones: A population-based study in China. Cancer Research. 2008;**68**:6442-6452

[18] Castro FA et al. Inflammatory gene variants and the risk of biliary tract cancers and stones: A population-based study in China. BMC Cancer. 2012;**12**:468

[19] Srivastava A et al. CCR5 Delta32 polymorphism: Associated with gallbladder cancer susceptibility. Scandinavian Journal of Immunology. 2008;**67**:516-522

[20] Sharma KL et al. Association of liver X receptors (LXRs) genetic variants to gallbladder cancer susceptibility. Tumour Biology. 2013;**34**:3959-3966

[21] Jiao X et al. hOGG1 Ser326Cys polymorphism and susceptibility to gallbladder cancer in a Chinese population. International Journal of Cancer. 2007;**121**:501-505

[22] Rege RV et al. Inflammation and a thickenedmucus layer inmice with cholesterol gallstones. The Journal of Surgical Research. 1998;**74**:81-85

[23] Lavoie B et al. Disruption of gallbladder smooth muscle function is an early feature in the development of cholesterol gallstone disease. Neurogastroenterology and Motility. 2012;**24**:e313-e324

[24] Maurer KJ. T-cell function is critical for murine cholesterol gallstone formation. Gastroenterology. 2007;**133**:1304-1315

[25] van Erpecum KJ et al. Gallbladder histopathology during murine gallstone formation: Relation to motility and concentrating function. Journal of Lipid Research. 2006;**47**:32-41

[26] Duarte I et al. Metaplasia and precursor lesions of gallbladder carcinoma. Frequency, distribution, and probability of detection in routine histologic samples. Cancer. 2013;**72**:1878-1884

[27] Mukhopadhyay S et al. A review of 400 routinely resected specimens. Archives of Pathology & Laboratory Medicine. 2015;**129**:386-390

[28] Mathur SK et al. Correlation of gallstone characteristics with mucosal changes in gall bladder. Tropical Gastroenterology. **2012;33**:39-44

[29] Sakamoto H et al. A close relationship between intestinal metaplasia and Cdx2 expression in human gallbladders with cholelithiasis. Human Pathology. 2007;**38**:66-71

[30] Regalo G et al. Hacking cell differentiation: Trerouting in reprogramming, lineage infidelity and metaplasia. EMBO Molecular Medicine. 2013;**5**:1154-1164

[31] Leong RW, Sung JJ. Specie Helicobacter e malattie epatobiliari. Alimentary Pharmacology Ecology. 2012;**16**:1037-1045

[32] Nagata E et al. The relation between carcinoma of the gallbladder and an anomalous connection between the choledochus and the pancreatic duct. Annals of Surgery. 1995;**202**(2):182-202

[33] Kobayashi S et al. Prophylactic excision of the gallbladder and bile duct for patients with pancreaticobiliary Maljunction. Archives of Surgery. 2011;**136**:759-763

[34] Funabiki T et al. Pancreaticobiliary maljunction and carcinogenesis to biliary and pancreatic malignancy. Langenbeck's Archives of Surgery. 2009;**394**:159-169

[35] Hanada K et al. Gene mutations of K-ras in gallbladder mucosae and gallbladder carcinoma with an anomalous junction of the pancreaticobiliary duct. The American Journal of Gastroenterology. 1999;**94**:1638-1642

[36] Matsubara T et al. K-ras point mutations in cancerous and noncancerous biliary epithelium in patients with pancreaticobiliary maljunction. Cancer. 1996;**77**:1752-1757

[37] Towfigh S et al. Porcelain Gallbladder Is Not Associated with Gallbladder Carcinoma: Southeeastern Surgical Congress. The American Surgeon; 2011

[38] Kim JH et al. Should we perform surgical management in all patients suspected porcelain gallbladder? Hepatogaastroenterology. 2009;**56**(93):943-945

[39] Park JY et al. Long term follow up of Gallbladder Polyps. Journal of Gastroenterological Hepatology. 2019;**24**(2):219-222

[40] Landgren AM et al. Autoimmune disease and subsequent risk of developing alimentary tract cancers among 4.5 million US male veterans. Cancer. 2011;**117**:1163-1171

[41] Joffe N et al. Primary carcinoma of the gallbladder associated with chronic inflammatory bowel disease. Clinical Radiology. 1991;**32**:319-324

[42] Buckles DC et al. In primary sclerosing cholangitis, gallbladder polyps are frequently malignant. The American Journal of Gastroenterology. 2012;**97**:1138-1142

[43] de Werra C et al. L'ittero ostruttivo quale sequela del Carcinoma della Colecisti. In: Atti del 109° Congresso SIC. 2007

[44] Hederstrom E et al. Ulthrasonography in carcinoma of the gallbladder: Diagnostic difficulties and pitfalls. Acta Radiologica. 1987;**28**:6

[45] Koga A et al. Ultrasonographic detection of early and curable carcinoma of the gallbladder. British Journal of Surgery. 1985;**72**:728-730

[46] Okamoto M et al. Ultrasonographic evidence of association of polyps and stones with gallbladder cancer. The American Journal of Gastoenterology. 2009;**94**(2):446-450

[47] Soiva M et al. Ultrasonography in carcinoma of the gallbladder. Acta Radiology. 1987;**28**(6):711-714

[48] de Werra C et al. Diagnostica nel sospetto ultrasonografico di Carcinoma della Colecisti. In: Atti del 104° Congresso SIC. 2002

[49] Albores-Saavedra J et al. Carinoembryonic antigen in normal, paraneoplastic and neoplastic gallbladder epithelium. Cancer. 1983;**52**:1069-1072

[50] Baskaran V. Value of CEA and AFP in the diagnosis and prognosis of carcinoma of the gallbladder. Tropical Gastroenterology. 2001;**22**(4):227-229

[51] Inui K, Nakazawa S. Diagnosis of depth of invasion of gallbladder carcinoma with endosonography. Nippon Geka Gakkai Zasshi. 1998;**99**(10):696-699

[52] Kimura K et al. Diagnosis of pT2 gallbladder cancer by serial examinations with endoscopic ultrasound and angiography. Journal of Gastroenterology. 2012;**37**(3):200-203

[53] Rendano F, Salfi R, de Werra C, Sarno A. Diagnostica pre-intra e post-operatoria dei tumori epatici. In: Atti del

IX Congresso Nazionale SICO. 1985. pp. 207-213

[54] Gadaleta A et al. Ultrasonography, computed tomography and transhepatic cholangiography in carcinoma of the gallbladder. RAYS (Roma). 1984;**9**(2):75-83

[55] Rendano F, Amorosa L, Borriello C, de Werra C. La diagnostica oncologica del fegato Atti dell'XI Congresso Nazionale SICO. Genova; 1987. pp. 1021-1028

[56] Koh T et al. Possibility of differential diagnosis of small polypoid lesions in the gallbladder using FDG-PET. Clinical Positron Imaging. 2010;**3**(5):213-218

[57] Shukla PJ et al. Does PET-CT scan have a role prior to radical re-resection for incidental gallbladder cancer. HPB: The Official Journal of the International Hepato Pancreato Biliary Association. 2008;**10**:439-445

[58] de Werra C et al. Diagnosi precoce del Carcinoma della Colecisti. In: Atti del 110° Congresso SIC. 2008

[59] Fong Y et al. Evidence-based gallbladder cancer staging: Changing cancer staging by analysis of data from the national cancer database. Annals of Surgery. 2016;**243**:767-774

[60] Nevin JE et al. Carcinoma of the gallbladder. Staging, treatement and prognosis. Cancer. 1976;**37**:141-148

[61] Available from: www.cancer.org/cancer/gallbladdercancer/detailedguide/gallbladder-staging

[62] AJCC Cancer Staging Manual. Seventh ed. New York: Springer-Verlag; 2010. Available from: www.cancerstaging.net

[63] Lamarca A, Galdy S, Barriuso J, McNamara MG, Hubner RA. Gallbladder cancer: Has the time come to move from late palliation to early intervention? Cancer Treatment Reviews. 2019;**82**:101925

[64] Sheth S, Bedford A. Malignant diseases of the gallbladder and biliary tree. Radiologic Clinics. 2019;**57**(2):409-424

[65] Turaga KK, Girotra M, Johnston FM. Gallbladder cancer: Surgical management. Current Problems in Surgery. 2019;**56**(3):100704

[66] Valle JW, Lamarca A, Goyal L, Barriuso J, Zhu AX, Galle PR. New horizons for precision medicine in biliary tract cancers. Cancer Discovery. 2020;**10**(3):343-355. DOI: 10.1158/2159-8290.CD-19-0681

[67] Shroff RT, Javle MM. Treatment of metastatic gallbladder cancer: New insights into an old disease. Current Oncology Reports. 2018;**20**(11):91. DOI: 10.1007/s11912-018-0737-4

[68] Lamarca A, Hubner RA, David Ryder W, Valle JW. Second-line chemotherapy in advanced biliary cancer: A systematic review. Annals of Oncology. 2014;**25**(12):2328-2338. DOI: 10.1093/annonc/mdu258

[69] de Werra P et al. The role of Laproscopic Cholecystectomy in incidental gallbladder carcinoma. In: 12th International Congress of the European Association for Endoscopic Surgery. 2004

[70] Goyal G, Philip PA. Role of immune checkpoint inhibition in the treatment of biliary tract cancer. Journal of Gastrointestinal Oncology;**9**(1):139-143. DOI: 10.21037/jgo.2017.10.01

[71] Kanthan R, Senger JL, Ahmed S. Gallbladder cancer in the 21st century. Journal of Oncology. 2014;**2015**